D1061373

POLICY ANALYSIS:

INTRODUCTION AND APPLICATIONS TO HEALTH PROGRAMS

POLICY ANALYSIS:

INTRODUCTION AND APPLICATIONS TO HEALTH PROGRAMS

by
MARVIN R. BURT
Burt Associates, Incorporated

INFORMATION RESOURCES PRESS/WASHINGTON, D.C./1974 I^R_P

RA 427
B9

Fairleigh Dickinson
University Library

Teaneck, New Jersey

Copyright © 1974 by Information Resources Press,
a division of Herner & Company.
All Rights Reserved.
Printed in the United States of America.

No part of this publication may be reproduced, stored in a retrieval system, or trans-
mitted, in any form or by any means, electronic, mechanical, photocopying, recording,
or otherwise, without the prior written permission of the publisher.

Available from
Information Resources Press
2100 M Street, N.W.
Washington, D.C. 20037

Library of Congress Catalog Card Number 74-81587

ISBN 0-87815-013-7

4/19/79 $16.00

PREFACE

For some time now, persons seeking information on how to conduct a policy analysis have had to struggle through collections of readings, each of which usually reflects the author's particular experiences in conducting his version of policy analysis. There has not been available a brief, convenient guide to introduce the student or practitioner to the methodologies for conducting a policy analysis. This lack, coupled with the frustrations my students and I experienced in attempting to communicate these concepts and techniques during a new course which I developed at The George Washington University, led to this book.

Essentially, this book is intended as an introduction to the application of policy analysis, but should prove useful to practitioners as a guide to the conduct of a policy analysis. Although the material is presented in sufficient generality to include most program analyses, the specific examples are of health program analysis as practiced by health planners and program analysts.

Some aspects of policy analysis are not discussed in this brief document, including the organization and structure of service delivery systems, and political and bureaucratic considerations. The discussions, intentionally, tend to be mechanistic, to enable the reader to proceed sequentially through the essential steps of the analysis process.

Because the focus is on policy analysis methodologies, various other aspects of policy analysis are not fully considered. First, the broader conceptual framework for policy analysis and government decision making is not emphasized. This is discussed in several of the books and articles listed in the bibliography (notably, in Yehezkel Dror's *Public Policymaking Re-examined*).

Second, although policy analysis may be considered within the context of PPB (Planning-Programming-Budgeting), the structural and information system aspects of PPB are not discussed. More about this may be found in several publications listed in the bibliography (notably, in David Novick's *Program Budgeting*).

Third, many of the models of choice in decision theory are ignored. I have intentionally chosen to emphasize a rational model, with the principal criterion of choice being efficiency. Many other criteria—of an administrative, political, or other nature—are not discussed. Again, several items listed in the bibliography can be consulted for more information on these criteria. I have found Bauer and Gergen's *The Study of Policy Formulation* to be a useful, brief overview of the major schools of thought (particularly Chapters 1, 2, and 3).

Fourth, the application of policy analysis to social programs is emphasized. I have chosen to focus exclusively on health programs in order to provide a consistent framework for the discussion. I could just as easily have chosen another or several other types of programs, because, although the focus is on health, the approach is generally applicable to other programs as well.

Part I of this book describes the process of conducting a policy analysis, using examples to emphasize and clarify. Part II presents three cases in which policy analysis has been successfully employed. The first two cases analyze alternative future courses of action in maternal and child health services and in emergency ambulance services. The third case is an after-the-fact evaluation of a family planning program. These cases are not intended to represent perfection, but, nevertheless, may be regarded as examples of good analyses. All three of the cases meet the most important criterion of success for policy analysis—each had an important influence on policy.

This book has benefited from comments provided by Philip Reeves and Steven Chitwood of The George Washington University and by Harold Adams of the State University of New York at Albany. I am also grateful to the students in my course, Urban Analysis, who provided useful feedback on an earlier draft of this book. Of course, I must bear the sole responsibility for the final product.

WASHINGTON, D.C.

FEBRUARY 1974

ACKNOWLEDGEMENTS

Figure 1 is reprinted by kind permission of The RAND Corporation. Table 4, Figure 8, and three paragraphs appearing on pages 42, 43, and 44 are reprinted by kind permission of *Operations Research*.

CONTENTS

Part I

Methodology

CHAPTER 1

INTRODUCTION

Definition of Policy Analysis

Policy analysis is neither a single method nor a collection of methods and techniques. Because policy analyses derive their character largely from the problems they address, they may seem to bear little resemblance to each other. Also, the specific tools or analytical techniques may differ from study to study, because the problems addressed and the questions asked about various policies and programs are different. What then is policy analysis?

Policy analysis is a practical philosophy on how to assist a decision maker with complex problems of choice under conditions of uncertainty. As it is presented in this book, policy analysis can be characterized as a systematic approach to helping a decision maker choose a course of action by investigating his entire problem, searching out alternatives, and comparing these alternatives in the light of their consequences, using an analytic framework to bring expert judgment and intuition to bear on the problem.

Policy analysis is intended to be an alternative or supplement to the more traditional methods of decision making based on incrementalism, intuitive judgment, and trial and error methods of operation. It is characterized by a systematic approach encompassing: the definition of the problem or issue in question; the statement of government objectives and criteria by which the achievement of those objectives can be measured; the consideration of alternative programs or policies for achieving those objectives; and the selection of the preferred alternatives, based upon the evaluation criteria and consideration of other factors, including political constraints and feasibility.[1]

Governments have been conducting crude policy analyses for some time. Indeed, incrementalism itself is a crude form of policy analysis, focusing upon means rather than on ends and upon changes in the prevailing course

---

[1] For an excellent discussion of the political feasibility issue, see Arnold J. Meltsner, "Political Feasibility and Policy Analysis," *Public Administration Review, 32*(6):859–867, December 1972.

of action rather than on a broader spectrum of alternatives. What is changing is the new emphasis upon a more systematic method of analysis, focusing on ends and outputs and their relationship to inputs rather than on inputs only. It is this focus that most clearly differentiates policy analysis from more traditional methods of analysis.

Concepts

Policy analysis, in one form or another, has been with us for some time— particularly as applied to military problems. Although a great deal has been learned during that time about conducting such analyses, it has not been sufficient to supply a sequence of steps or rules that, if followed mechanically, would automatically guarantee good analyses, because, to some extent, policy analysis is more of an art form rather than an exact science. Unlike physical chemistry or statistics, for example, it is not a body of knowledge and skills that can be acquired without becoming involved in particular applications.

The analysis must contain subjective judgments, and some uncertainties will be encountered. These have to be carefully considered and documented. Therefore, a discussion of how analysis is accomplished must be limited to indicating some guidelines, principles, and illustrative examples.

THE SCIENTIFIC METHOD

The core of policy analysis is the scientific method. The use of this method distinguishes policy analysis from other types of studies intended to support the decision-making process.[2] In a methodological sense, we try to be as scientific as possible in the conduct of the analysis. Usually, the scientific method implies the presence, in some form, of the following stages:

Formulation: Defining the issues of concern, clarifying the objectives, and limiting the problems.

---

[2] This is not intended to suggest that this method is not and has not been used in the past to varying degrees; but traditional government studies are characterized by a lack of application of the scientific method.

Search: Determining the relevant data and seeking alternative programs of action to resolve the issues.

Explanation: Building a model and using it to explore the consequences of the alternative programs, usually by obtaining estimates of their cost and performance.

Interpretation: Deriving the conclusions and indicating a preferred alternative or course of action. This may be a combination of features from previously considered alternatives or their modification to reflect factors not taken into account earlier.

Verification: Testing the conclusion by experimentation. It is rarely possible, however, to carry out this step until a program is implemented. A program plan should call for evaluations which can provide after-the-fact verification.

Figure 1 depicts the flow of the preceding activities during a policy analysis.

FORMULATION

At this first stage of analysis, it is necessary to isolate the questions or issues involved, to establish the context within which these issues are to be addressed, to clarify the objectives and the criteria by which their attainment is to be measured, and to identify and state the relationships among the important variables. These relationships among variables may not be well understood, particularly where empirical knowledge is scant; however, even where hypothetical relationships are identified, the process will help to make the structure of the analysis more clear.

Formulation may be regarded as the most important stage of analysis. It identifies the *real* problem that is to be addressed and points the way toward a solution. In a very complex problem, a large proportion of the total time and resources available to conduct the analysis may be expended during this stage.

A principal objective of the formulation stage is to consider what is most meaningful and significant to the decision maker, that is, the client. A frequent mistake is to accept fully the client's original statement of what is wanted and how he perceives his problem. When this occurs, the analyst may set about building a model and gathering information without ade-

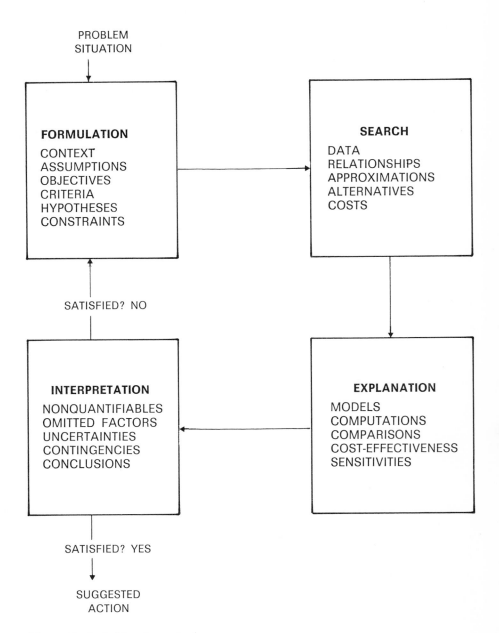

Figure 1. Activities in analysis.

Source: E. S. Quade, ed. *Analysis for Military Decisions.* Santa Monica, Calif., The RAND
      Corporation, 1964. p. 158.

quately considering and identifying the actual problem and without determining whether the answer will contribute significantly to alleviating the problem. The author has *never* conducted a policy analysis that finally considered the problem as originally stated by the decision maker.

For example, a decision maker may decide that his problem is determining where to place a comprehensive health center. During the formulation stage, the analyst may find instead that the real problem is how to provide outpatient health services to meet the demands or needs of low-income citizens. The best way to accomplish this might be by building a single Neighborhood Health Center (or several), or by providing services through other delivery mechanisms (for example, improved hospital outpatient departments, group practices, etc.). Similarly, if the decision maker's principal concern is not in providing health services per se, but, rather, in reducing certain indexes of health morbidity, mortality, and disability, a comprehensive health service program may not be his most viable alternative. Perhaps programs focusing specifically upon the maternal and child health services should be considered (if his principal concern is in reducing the infant mortality rate), or early case-finding and screening of chronic handicapping conditions (if his principal concern is handicapping conditions among children). Some of these trade-offs are very well-described in the case cited in Chapter 4.

SEARCH

This phase of policy analysis is concerned with finding the alternatives to be considered and the data or evidence on which the analysis is to be based. One alternative is to do nothing (that is, continue with the present course of action). The essence of policy analysis, however, is a consideration of alternatives to an existing or proposed course of action. Frequently, data are hard to come by. The availability of data on the health status of the population in particular communities, for example, varies considerably among communities. Some have initiated ongoing community health surveys, while others have very little data. It is also very difficult to determine what the impact of proposed alternatives might be.

For these reasons, policy analysis may have to depend upon informed judgment to a considerable degree. Theoretically, the search for data can be endless, and it is almost impossible to completely eliminate the uncertainties in most analysis problems. Nearly every study will have limitations on the time and resources within which it must be completed. The analyst, therefore, must exercise judicious judgment to determine when the data-gathering phase should be cut off. Unfortunately, a common pitfall of many studies is that the data-gathering phase consumes so much of the available time and resources that very little analysis is actually conducted.

EXPLANATION (EVALUATION)

The use of a model or a set of models can be an important vehicle for choosing among alternatives. Ideally, models provide mechanisms for estimating or predicting the consequences of each alternative. The role of the model is to provide a means of obtaining costs and performance or output estimates for each alternative. On rare occasions, a fairly elaborate computer program may combine most or all of the various factors needed to determine the costs and outputs of each alternative. More commonly, however, the subjects and criteria are too complex for the use of a single model. Rarely, in policy analysis, is it possible to determine a clearly optimum solution. For many complex problems, it is not possible to build quantitative or even very formalized models.

Frequently, the most valuable function of a model is explanatory; in other words, to organize our thinking. This may be as simple as a schematic flowchart depicting the process followed in a particular treatment program, or it may consist of a schematic drawing showing the relationships between the various elements of a health system in a community. Considerations for building such models are discussed in Chapter 3.

Rarely is the first model developed in the course of analysis the final choice. Model building is an iterative process. As a study goes on, models are refined, eliminated, replaced, etc. Models may change because of a better understanding of the questions being asked. For example, it may be determined that the original impression of the structure of the community health system was quite wrong and that, during the investigation, it was discovered that the various elements had entirely different relationships to each other.

INTERPRETATION

Here, the analyst attempts to interpret his work. An important element in this stage of analysis, as well as in previous stages, is to involve—in addition to the sponsor or decision maker—persons with substantive expertise in the field being studied. For example, it would be very difficult to foresee how many of the pitfalls encountered in interpreting health system data could be avoided without the participation of some health practitioners. At this stage, it is entirely possible that a decision could be made to recycle and reformulate the problem. It could be that the desirable alternatives are completely infeasible and that further analysis has to be conducted to develop more feasible alternatives. In considering the feasibility of implementing alternatives, the political process becomes paramount. If policy analysis is to be something more than an intellectual abstraction, and if its primary purpose is to influence policy, then it must consider the political realities.

Whether the analysis should present conclusions and recommendations is a subject of some debate among policy analysts. Clearly, it is important for the user of the analysis to be able to distinguish between what the study actually shows and the analyst's recommendations, based upon what the analyst believes the study implies. Therefore, the presentation of conclusions and recommendations is an important obligation of the policy analyst and may, in fact, be the most important contribution that he makes. It is important, however, that the recommendations and conclusions be clearly supported by the analysis.

Ultimately, the decision maker must exercise his own intuition and judgment in making the final decision; it is his responsibility and cannot be delegated to the analyst. The analyst, in conducting his analysis, can never completely consider all of the important factors and constraints that are involved. The decision maker may have political constraints, he may have his own interpretation of the data, or he may have completely different sources of information to draw upon.

VERIFICATION

Verification entails testing the conclusion by experimentation. This frequently is not possible to accomplish. Ideally, when a program is approved for implementation, a method of evaluation should be designed to determine the extent to which its goals are achieved. The evaluation should provide the feedback data necessary to verify the conclusions. The following general questions should be answered: How accurate are the effectiveness measures projected in the policy analysis? How accurate are the projected costs? To what extent are the goals achieved?

The case discussed in Chapter 6 is an evaluation that verifies the efficacy of a policy decision to embark on an extensive family planning program for American Indians.

Elements of a Policy Analysis

There are certain elements that are common to any policy analysis, irrespective of the subject matter.[3] These are:

The objective (or objectives): Policy analysis is undertaken for the purpose of suggesting, or helping to choose, a course of action which, in turn, must have an objective or aim. Policies or strategies are then examined and compared, based upon how efficiently and effectively they can accomplish the objective.

The alternatives: The different programs or means by which the objective or objectives can be attained.

The costs: Each alternative requires the use of specific quantities of resources which, once committed, cannot be used for other purposes.

A model (or models): A representation of the situation under study designed to predict the resource inputs into a system, the effectiveness outputs and, ideally, their relationships to each alternative. It is an abstraction of the relevant characteristics of the situation.[4]

A criterion (or criteria): Rules or tests for the selection of one alternative over another. These provide a method for ordering the alternatives, using their costs, and measuring their effectiveness.

---

[3] These are derived from Roland N. McKean, *Efficiency in Government Through Systems Analysis*, New York, John Wiley & Sons, Inc., 1958; and David Novick, ed., *Program Budgeting: Program Analysis and the Federal Government*, Cambridge, Mass., Harvard University Press, 1965.

[4] The means used to represent this abstraction may vary from a set of mathematical equations or a computer program to an idealized or actual description of the process or situation in which judgment alone is used to assess the consequences of various choices. In health policy analysis, the models often are closer to the latter end of the spectrum than to the former.

Guidelines for Conducting a Program Analysis[5]

Using the preceding elements of a program analysis as a base, the guidelines hereafter discussed should be followed in conducting a program analysis. (These are followed in considerable detail in Chapters 2 and 3.)

Structuring of the problem, design of the analysis, and the conceptual framework. The correct questions must be asked, and the problem must be properly structured. The objectives of the policies and programs must be clearly stated in policy terms, the relevant population must be defined, and the alternatives for evaluation must be selected. The two principal approaches are: the *fixed output approach*, wherein, for a specified level of output, the analyst attempts to attain the output at the lowest possible economic cost; and the *fixed budget approach*, wherein the analyst attempts to determine which alternatives (or combinations thereof) are likely to produce the highest output within the given budget level.[6] Several budget levels may be used to examine the sensitivity of the ranking of the alternatives to the output or budget levels.

Building the Model. The critical points are as follows:

1. Model building is an art—an experimental and iterative process.
2. The main purpose of building models is to develop a set of relationships among the objectives, the relevant alternatives available for obtaining them, and the estimated cost and output for each alternative.
3. The analyst must include the relevant factors and judiciously suppress those that are relatively unimportant.
4. The model must treat uncertainty.
5. The assumptions upon which the model is based must be made explicit.

TREATMENT OF UNCERTAINTY

Uncertainty must be treated explicitly. There are two types of uncertainty: uncertainty about the state of the world in the future, and statistical uncertainty or risk. The latter is usually less troublesome to handle. The former

---

[5] These are based primarily on: Gene Fisher, in: Novick, *Program Budgeting*, Chap. 3.
[6] In a good analysis, both methods should be tested alternatively.

is most often handled by techniques of sensitivity analysis.[7] For example, the analyst's best estimate could be that a program of improved maternal and infant health care would reduce the number of infant deaths in a community by 15. Due to uncertainties caused by a lack of relevant data on the effectiveness of such programs, however, the reduction could be from 12 to 17. In the case discussed in Chapter 4, the analyst uses the 12 to 17 range to express this uncertainty and to determine how sensitive the results are to this variation.

In sensitivity analysis, if there are key parameters about which the analyst is uncertain, he may use several values (perhaps high, medium, and low), rather than only the one which be believes is most nearly accurate, to determine how sensitive the results (the ranking of alternatives being considered) are to the variations in uncertain parameters.

FUTURE YEAR COSTS

Two factors must be considered in estimating future year costs: inflation (causing costs to rise) and the economic concept that the value of a dollar in future years should be discounted (causing costs to decline). For example, next year it might cost $1,050[8] to purchase an item of equipment now costing $1,000. An economist, however, would say that next year's costs should be discounted and that the present value of the $1,050 expenditure is only $955.[9] This apparent dilemma is further discussed in Chapter 3.

VALIDITY CHECKING

This relates to validating the accuracy of the model. A controlled experiment is rarely possible for validating the accuracy of the model, but may be

[7] Contingency analysis and *a fortiori* analysis are less commonly used. In contingency analysis, the question is how the ranking of alternatives holds up when a change in criteria for evaluating alternatives is postulated or a major change in general environment is assumed. *A fortiori* analysis may be used when the analyst feels that the intuitively acceptable dominant alternative X might be a poor choice when compared to alternative Y. In comparing the two, the analyst may deliberatively resolve the major uncertainties in favor of X to see how it compares under adverse conditions. If Y still appears favorable, there is a very strong case in its favor. For examples of contingency analysis and *a fortiori* analysis, see E.S. Quade and W. J. Boucher, *Systems Analysis and Policy Planning*, Santa Monica, Calif., The RAND Corporation, 1968.

[8] This assumes a 5-percent rate of inflation.

[9] The formula used is $\dfrac{1}{(1 + r)^n}$ or $\dfrac{\$1,050}{(1 + 10)^1} = \$955$ at a 10-percent discount rate (r) for one year (n). Rates between 5 to 20 percent have been proposed.

possible after-the-fact. It may be possible to validate the model using a roughly analogous existing situation. The critical questions here are whether the model can describe known facts and situations reasonably well, and whether it can assign causes to known effects.[10] The model will not be useful unless the analyst and others find it persuasive.

QUALITATIVE SUPPLEMENTATION
This may take several forms:

1. Qualitative analysis per se as an integral part of the total analytical effort.
2. Interpretation of the quantitative work.
3. Discussion of relevant nonquantitative considerations that could not be taken into account in the formal analysis.

Conclusion

The discussion of methodologies appropriate for program analysis began with the scientific method and proceeded to successively lower levels of abstraction, to the point where the preceding relatively definitive guidelines were proposed. These guidelines conform essentially to the activities in analysis depicted in Figure 1.

[10] Gene Fisher, in: Novick, *Program Budgeting*, Chap. 3, would add the following questions: "When the principal parameters involved are varied, do the results remain consistent and plausible?"; "Can it handle special cases in which we already have some indications as to what the outcome should be?" Quade et al., *Systems Analysis and Policy Planning*, Introduction, noted that verifying the accuracy of the model is rarely possible.

CHAPTER 2

STRUCTURING THE PROBLEM, DESIGNING THE ANALYSIS, AND DEVELOPING THE CONCEPTUAL FRAMEWORK

The fundamental point discussed in this chapter is that the analyst must ask the right questions and focus the analysis upon answering them. It is in the design stage of analysis that most policy analysts either flounder hopelessly or move on toward success.

What are the right questions? There are no scientific guidelines to follow, therefore each analysis will usually require different questions.

The Analytical Structure

In conducting a policy analysis, a schematic diagram of the steps in the analytical process, showing the flow and relationships between each major step, can be of significant benefit to the analyst, as well as to the technical reviewer of the analysis. Figure 2 depicts such a schematic diagram as it applies to the major steps of any policy analysis, and it describes the major steps to be followed in our discussion. The process actually is more iterative than depicted in the simplified diagrams shown in Figures 1 and 2. Any stage may require returning to a previous stage to re-examine some elements.

In conducting an analysis of health programs, a schematic diagram such as that depicted in Figure 3 may be useful. In this case, health objectives, influenced by the characteristics of the health system, health status, and universe of need (the population requiring the services), determine the demand for health care. Other ways of meeting the demand are then defined in terms of alternative health programs, services (within the programs), and delivery vehicles (mechanisms for delivering the services).[1] These alternatives are influenced by various constraints; therefore, a mix of

---

[1] These will be explained in some detail later in this chapter.

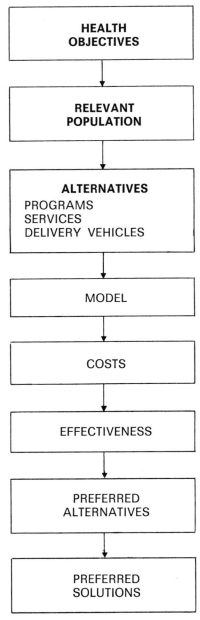

Figure 2. General analytical structure for health program analysis.

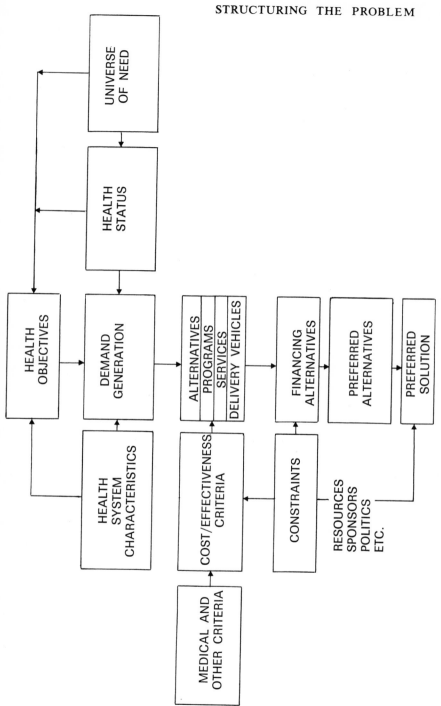

Figure 3. Analysis of alternatives.

criteria (cost-effectiveness, health, etc.), rather than one best criterion, usually is used to derive alternatives. Various financing mechanisms are then considered, and the preferred alternative programs, services, and delivery vehicles are determined. Finally, the preferred solution, in terms of a proposed program, is derived.

Definition of Objectives

The questions to be asked in an analysis are strongly dependent upon the objectives defined for the programs and conversely. Thus, in the analysis of social programs, in which objectives are not often clearly stated, the definition of objectives becomes particularly important. Analysis should be conducted at the highest level at which the components of a system share objectives; but the interaction of multiple, interacting objectives is so complex at this level that meaningful analysis becomes impossible. Indeed, a useful generalization is that the higher level the objective, the more difficult analysis becomes. Thus, suboptimization is necessary in order for analysis to be possible.

This means essentially that one proceeds to successively lower-level objectives until they are sufficiently discrete and the problem sufficiently manageable so that meaningful analysis is possible. For example, it is analytically impossible to consider social welfare as an objective. It is too diffuse and unmanageable analytically. Health, a subset of social welfare, is more discrete, but still is not manageable analytically. Only when health is further subdivided into definable objectives does the level become sufficiently low to be manageable analytically.

Now, if we measure the extent to which particular policies or programs achieve these health objectives, we are not only ignoring nonhealth, social welfare objectives, but we could be ignoring some health objectives that we have not included or measured. Thus, we have suboptimized because some aspects are ignored (or held constant). The trick is to accomplish this judiciously so that the ranking of alternatives is not sensitive to it. For example, health analyses (and those illustrated in this book are not exceptions) typically ignore how people believe they feel or their personal concept of healthiness. This could be affected by such factors as the attractiveness of the setting in which health services are offered, the clients' feelings of self-worth, etc. By ignoring these, is the analyst being judicious?

HEALTH OBJECTIVES

In health policy analysis, the preceding general guidelines might be operationalized by examining what is meant by health, by defining subcategories and objectives for it, and by relating them to the analytical context required for policy analysis.

Figure 4 depicts a hierarchy of health objectives. At the highest level is a general SOCIAL WELFARE objective. At the next level are subobjectives relating to EDUCATION, HEALTH, and OTHER. It was noted previously that, in order for meaningful analysis to be possible, lower level objectives had to be considered. The following are proposed for health programs:

To Improve Health Status: Expressed in terms of morbidity, mortality, and other indicators of ill health, such as disability days and work-loss days.

To Improve Health Care: Expressed in terms of requirements (demand) for various types of health services for the individual, the community, etc. This objective usually is expressed in terms of quantities of health services (for example, number of persons served by comprehensive health care, number of physician visits, etc.).

To Decrease the Health Gap: Basically derived from improved health status and health care. This objective is expressed in terms of differences in health status, receipt of health care, and health expenditures between groups of persons or communities in the society (for example, between the poor and nonpoor). While the first two types of objectives are absolute, this type is relative, focusing on the differences.

To Improve Health Related Factors: This objective recognizes that health programs are aimed at other welfare objectives, such as the reduction of poverty, psychic needs (which may include feeling well), and the desire to change existing institutions in terms of their attitudes toward clients and to promote more efficient and higher quality health care.

These four types of objectives are not independent, but rather overlap to a significant extent. Although health status and health care may be considered independently, health status usually is considered the primary determining factor that influences the demand for health care. Health gap objectives basically are derived from differentials among various segments of the population in health status and the receipt of health services. Health related objectives tend to form a separate dimension that relates to all of the other three.

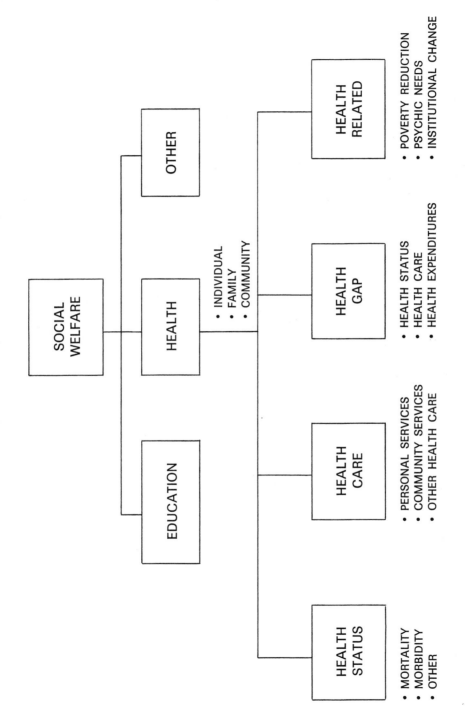

Figure 4. Health objectives.

HEALTH STATUS

Overall health objectives perhaps can best be expressed as the relative existence or nonexistence of ill health. The search for a universally applicable measure of ill health, however, has not been very fruitful. Certainly a composite index[2] that could measure the utility of alternative programs does not exist. Previously, indices of crude morbidity and mortality rates have been used. Death rates in the United States have been relatively constant since 1956; thus, greater attention has been paid to morbidity. The evaluation of morbidity and mortality rates is subject to much interpretation, as increased morbidity is often the result of reduced mortality (for example, the increased longevity of diabetics has increased morbidity while reducing mortality).[3]

Sullivan[4] has suggested four categories for classifying morbidity: confined, limited mobility, limited activity, and restricted activity; Chiang[5] has proposed an index comprising age-specific components derived from the death rate and from the incidence and duration of illness; Saunders[6] has suggested measuring health rather than illness, using a concept of individual functional adequacy to fulfill a social role; the U.S. Public Health Service[7] has experimented with a Q Theory, which essentially is an unweighted index summing morbidity and mortality by disease category; and Burt et al.[8] used four proxy indicators of health status—by age and sex—to demonstrate differences between the poor and nonpoor: one or more chronic conditions, restricting acute conditions, restricted activity days, and bed disability days.

The basic problem with using health status objectives is that there are great uncertainties in estimating the relationships between provision of

---

[2] The essential criteria to be met by such an index is that it be sensitive to the effectiveness of health programs and that it be composed of measurable components. This lack of a composite index is found in all social programs. See A. H. Packer, "Applying Cost-Effectiveness Concepts to the Community Health System," *Operations Research, 16*(2):237, March–April 1968.

[3] *Ibid.*

[4] National Center for Health Statistics. *Conceptual Problems in Developing an Index of Health.* Washington, D.C., U.S. Government Printing Office, 1965. U.S. Public Health Service Publication No. 1,000, Series 2, No. 17.

[5] National Center for Health Statistics. *An Index of Health—Mathematical Models.* Washington, D.C., U.S. Government Printing Office, 1965. U.S. Public Health Service Publication No. 1,000, Series 2, No. 5.

[6] B. S. Saunders. "Measuring Community Health Levels." *American Journal of Public Health, 54*(4):1063–1070, April 1964.

[7] U.S. Department of Health, Education, and Welfare. *International Classification of Diseases, Adapted for Use in the U.S.* 8th Rev. Washington, D.C., U.S. Government Printing Office, 1969.

[8] Marvin R. Burt et al., *Delivery and Financing of Health Services to the Poor: A Cost-Effectiveness Analysis.* Bethesda, Md., Resource Management Corp., 1967.

health services and achievement of some predictable (even probabilistic) impact on morbidity and mortality. A particularly critical problem is that as one considers comprehensive health care objectives, measures of health status tend to be relatively less meaningful.[9] Using available health status criteria, it cannot now be proven that comprehensive health care is better than noncomprehensive health care,[10] due to the lack of meaningful data.

To conclude this discussion of health status objectives, it seems appropriate to cite from *Delivery and Financing of Health Services to the Poor: A Cost-Effectiveness Analysis*:

> Ideally, a measure or set of measures should fully describe the properties of the goal. Occasionally, in health programs, this may be readily done. For example, if a program goal were to eliminate poliomyelitis from a community, the incidence of its occurrence could be checked year-by-year, and the costs of various program alternatives having this common goal could be compared. However, most of the epidemiological measures for which data are readily obtainable, and which have been used in public health in the past, are not directly relevant to the personal health goals of the nation in the 1970's. With a shift of emphasis away from specific disease control to comprehensive care, and the promotion of individual well-being, disagreement arises over what, given the state-of-the-art, could be included and quantified as benefits, as well as frustration over what should, but cannot be included (given the state-of-the-art). In addition, there is little agreement as to how one should handle intangible but highly important health benefits such as relief of pain, mental anguish, etc., to say nothing of such social benefits as increased employment, decreased divorce rates, etc.[11]

HEALTH CARE

The use of health care objectives, such as Provision of Family Planning Services to "X" Women, considerably simplifies the analysis while making it more useful to the decision maker, as this type of objective more closely

[9] Comprehensive health care is not well-defined. It is a relative term which suggests that, to the maximum extent possible, health services should be offered in one location (or in as few locations as possible), should be preventive (rather than episodic), and should be family oriented. The focus, therefore, is less upon the treatment or prevention of a specific disease or upon offering services to a particular type of client—as in a cancer clinic, for example—than it is upon offering a whole range of services which address a whole spectrum of health.

[10] The author has searched in vain for such evidence. The only meaningful study found little (if any) difference in health status between groups of persons subjected to each alternative. (See the Cornell Welfare Project, in: Burt et al., *Delivery and Financing of Health Services to the Poor*, p. 89.)

[11] Cornell Welfare Project. In: Burt et al. *Delivery and Financing of Health Services to the Poor*, p. 88.

reflects the real world in which demand for health services is an exogenous variable. This objective also reflects the current thrust of medical programs which emphasize comprehensive, preventive care rather than concentrating upon more specific dysfunctions. Health care objectives suffer from the disadvantage of circumventing the issue of improving health status, although they might be used in conjunction with health status objectives, as was done in the aforementioned analysis. The health status effectiveness measures used cannot fully reflect the total impact of the expenditures, nor, indeed, can any other measures do so; large expenditures for health programs have very little to do with reducing morbidity and mortality rates. We will see in Chapter 4 that a large part of comprehensive maternal and child health care programs have little impact on health status measures, because many of the health services are used for well-baby care, treatment of respiratory infections, etc. These services might have considerable impact on individual feelings of healthiness and meet professional service standards, but have little impact on health status. The use of health care objectives simplifies the analysis, as one can avoid—at least temporarily—the problem of measuring the change in health status that is attributable to the provision of health services to a group of persons. It is assumed that the objectives are the provision of higher levels of health service per se; the principal question then is what would be the relative efficiency of alternative means for providing these services.

HEALTH GAP

Health gap objectives are relative measures derived from health status or health care objectives. They specify the differences in health status and the receipt of health services between groups or communities in the society. They frequently involve considerations of equity, as in comparisons of health status between the poor and nonpoor.

A health gap objective can be measured in terms of health status, health services (health care), or some combination of the two. For example, the gap can be measured by the difference in health status and/or health service between the poor and nonpoor.

The following indicators of health status have been used to define the gap: limitations of activity due to chronic conditions; frequency of hospitalization and length of stay; incidence of chronic illness by type—heart conditions, mental and nervous conditions, arthritis and rheumatism, high blood pressure, orthopedic impairments, and visual impairments (these were not age-adjusted); one or more chronic conditions, chronic conditions causing activity limitations, number of restricted-activity days, and number of bed-disability days; school-loss days and work-loss days; mortality rates, utilization rates in terms of doctor visits, and personal health expenditures and insurance coverage.[12] Objectives can be expressed by eliminating or narrowing the health gaps.

HEALTH RELATED FACTORS

Health related objectives include: reducing the incidence of poverty, meeting psychic needs of persons as they relate to health care and mental health, achieving changes in existing institutions and organizations, helping the poor to maintain their self-respect, ensuring that they actually use existing facilities when the need arises, ascertaining that facilities are located in neighborhoods where they are easily accessible, and ensuring that no racial or class discrimination exists in the provision of health services. Health related objectives also include the use of health programs as vehicles for community organization and involvement, for developing manpower training and employment opportunities for the poor, for reorganizing and reforming health institutions and the attitudes of health personnel, and for cooperating with nonhealth agencies.

The task of defining meaningful, measurable goals and objectives for health programs is made considerably more difficult by the varied concepts of comprehensive health care and the advocacy of positive as opposed to negative goals. These concepts can have a considerable impact upon the demand for health services.

The movement toward positive goals is expressed by Richard Lichtman:[13]

The change from a social system that acts to eliminate disease to one whose function is the promotion of health is part of a revolution in man's account

---

[12] See Burt et al., *Delivery and Financing of Health Services to the Poor*, Chapters 2, 3, and 4. The essential purpose of this gap analysis was to demonstrate the difference in health status and the receipt of health services between the poor and nonpoor.

[13] As quoted in a study directed by Ron Burlage of the Institute for Policy Studies. *New York Municipal Hospitals: A Policy Review*. Washington, D.C., 1967, p. A-62.

of himself, all of whose ramifications cannot be comprehended. What it signifies, in part at least, is that man has become so capable of altering the world about him and his relationship to it that he need no longer tolerate as the definition of illness and its avoidance those conditions that seem indigenous to a prior age. It may once have been a supreme achievement to avoid illness but the task of culture now is to engender health.

Lichtman's ideas are reflected in the growing professional and social concern with continuous comprehensive health care, which is based on the concept that health is a continuing need. If one accepts this concept of health requirements for the population, there are basically two ways of estimating it: first, by estimating need, using the health status data and seeking medical opinion to translate it into health services; and second, by accepting demand as an exogenously determined variable, using historical data on utilization of health services as a basis for measuring it.[14] In the latter case, the utilization rate for upper- or middle-income persons might be used to derive more adequate rates for the poor. The estimation of need is extremely difficult:[15]

Scientific standards of need are debatable and debated. They cannot be drawn without balancing the effects and the benefits of the service against the cost of providing it. Does one *need* annual checkups, semiannual, monthly, or weekly ones? Does one *need* to speed recovery from a painful condition—and if so, how much? Does one *need* to spend time reassuring the patient? The greater the ability of medicine to aid the individual in matters not involving life or death (the greater the departure from what many would term an absolute), the more difficult it is to arrive at a consensus of need as contrasted with "could use" or "would be of some value."

One must, therefore, define a combination of health status and health care objectives constrained by a variety of health related objectives. The fact that all of these types of objectives are relevant in conducting health program analysis presents an analytical problem. The implications of this state vis-a-vis measures of effectiveness and costs will be discussed later, particularly in Chapters 3, 4, and 6.

---

[14] Unfortunately, demand is influenced by a variety of factors, such as the availability of service (the supply), the price to the consumer, economic status, and ethnicity. It is, therefore, a very weak reed to lean upon in estimating health service requirements.

[15] Rashi Fein. *The Doctor Shortage*. Washington, D.C., The Brookings Institution, 1967, p. 24.

Estimating the Relevant Population

As objectives expressed in social policy analysis are ultimately concerned with people, the relevant population must be estimated and projected to the last year of the planning period.[16]

Census data are the usual source of population estimates. Although complete counts are accomplished every 10 years, other surveys are often conducted during the interview periods. Projected population estimates also are frequently available.

A reasonably adequate technique is to estimate the population in a base year (say 1970) and, for the succeeding five-year interval (1970 to 1975), to estimate (by age group) the base-year population, deaths, births, and net migration. The algebraic sum of these elements yields the estimated population for 1975.[17] This is illustrated in Table 1. Similar techniques can be used to estimate the population of specific socioeconomic groups (for example, blacks, low-income persons, etc.). Because the demand for health services is quite sensitive to age, population projections should specify age groups.

Table 1.
Population Projection

Population (000)	*Year*					
	1970	*1971*	*1972*	*1973*	*1974*	*1975*
Initial Population						
Deaths (−)						
Births (+)						
Net Migration						
Total						

---

16 The significance of this procedure is illustrated by an analysis of programs serving low-income persons, which projected that the number of low-income persons would decline from 47.3 million in 1967 to 42.9 million in 1973. As 1973 was the last program year, 42.9 million was used as the universe of need—a reduction of 4.4 million clients.

17 A complete explanation of these procedures is contained in Robert C. Atchley, *Population Projections and Estimates for Local Areas.* Oxford, Scripps Foundation, 1970.

Selection and Evaluation of Alternatives

The selection of alternatives to be considered in the analysis depends strongly upon the desired objectives. The analyst's imagination, versatility, and knowledge of the health system are crucial. The advice of experts is particularly vital at this stage. Similar alternatives may already exist— perhaps in a distant city. Each alternative must be evaluated using a consistent set of objectives, costs, and output criteria. Existing programs should be included as alternatives. For example, if the objectives are to improve the health status and to increase the quantities of specific outpatient health services delivered to low-income persons in a city, the existing delivery mechanisms (for example, physicians operating in solo practice, hospital outpatient departments, etc.) should be evaluated. Other alternatives also should be evaluated (for example, comprehensive health centers, physicians in group practice, improved hospital outpatient departments, etc.) using comparable criteria. Examples of such a comparison are discussed in Chapter 3.

Similar techniques should be used when services contained in alternatives are not identified (for example, comprehensive health care for children, family planning, maternal and child health care, and dental care), as illustrated in Chapter 4.

3

BUILDING THE MODEL AND
CONDUCTING THE ANALYSIS

This chapter will concentrate on the remaining steps in program analysis: building the model, estimating program costs, measuring program effectiveness, treatment of uncertainty, discounting, qualitative supplementation, selecting the preferred alternatives, and determining the preferred solution.

Building the Model

Program analysis utilizes a model that is intended to represent the relationships between resource inputs (funds, personnel, facilities, etc.), alternative programs, and effectiveness (utility) outputs.[1] This may be expressed in the following simplified diagrammatical form:

INPUTS		OUTPUTS
Resources	**Programs**	**Effectiveness**
$, Personnel, etc.	1 . . . n	Objectives

The essential task of the analyst is to identify, for the decision maker, the mix and quantity of programs that will maximize the value of the system in question, subject to an assumed set of conditions (constraints). Budget constraints (or alternative budget constraints) may be a factor. If the budget is fixed, or alternative fixed levels are assumed, the analyst's objective will

---

[1] In operations research literature, many other model types are suggested and distinguished by such terms as "optimization and simulation" and "deterministic and stochastic," among others. A. H. Packer, "Applying Cost-Effectiveness Concepts to the Community Health System," *Operations Research,* 16(2):227–254, March–April 1968, suggests the terms "analytical," referring to models which attempt to determine optimum solutions, and "simulation," referring to models which use heuristic techniques and do not seek optimum solutions. For a considerably broader definition of models, see David W. Miller and Martin K. Starr, *Executive Decisions and Operations Research,* Englewood Cliffs, N.J., Prentice-Hall, 1965. Chapters 7, 8, and 13.

be to maximize effectiveness within the various constraints. At alternative budget levels, different configurations may maximize effectiveness. Various incremental combinations may be tested to determine whether the additional increments required to achieve effectiveness are worth the cost. The analysis should indicate the marginal cost-effectiveness of additional investments in alternatives and eliminate from consideration inferior alternatives —that is, system configurations dominated by alternatives that are either more effective and no more costly, or less expensive and no less effective.[2]

Estimating Program Costs

Program costs constitute the input side of the model. The costs of alternative medical care programs can be estimated in several ways:

1. The first method involves the development of a production function for medical services by determining the value of the factor inputs (for example, costs of equipment, floor space, medical equipment) and the average physician's annual net receipts; the total represents the cost of producing the medical services. This method is most useful for costing specific types of clinics, but is relatively difficult for costing physicians in private practice. A doctor's equipment inventory varies greatly, depending on his training, skills, and regional location; also on his location within a city. For example, the doctor with offices near a medical laboratory will have less laboratory equipment of his own than will the doctor with no nearby laboratory. While these problems may be overcome, they must be clearly recognized and accounted for.[3]

2. A second method requires a knowledge of the specific services that are needed by the client population in question. Fee schedules often are available, and these can be used to calculate the cost of supplying a particular mix of services. The problem in using this technique is that specific mixes of services usually are not precisely known.

2 For a more mechanistic and more traditional operations research definition of the task, see Packer, "Applying Cost-Effectiveness Concepts," p. 232. Various operations research models may be employed in addition to, or within, the cost-effectiveness model depicted above. Packer has suggested that, due to the stochastic nature of the health system, simulation models are the most applicable; *Ibid.*

3 For inpatient services, many factors of production are used jointly to provide more than one service. For example, costs of general services and overhead in hospitals are difficult to allocate to specific services.

3. A third method that has been used with some success is determining the cost of providing one average visit to a physician. This can be done by dividing the physician's gross annual receipts by the number of patient visits to arrive at a cost per patient visit. A major problem with this method is that all visits to physicians are lumped into one category. Nevertheless, it is a useful (but rather crude) way to determine costs of providing services. Adjustments may have to be made to account for different types of patients.

4. Few medical programs that are now being proposed have not been tried somewhere previously. Cost (and perhaps effectiveness) data from these existing programs often can be used to estimate the cost of similar programs elsewhere. Adjustments usually have to be made to account for differences such as salaries, types of patients served, location, and types and extensiveness of the services offered. It is particularly important to define, in some detail, specifically what services are offered by the program. For example, there are many possible versions of comprehensive health centers, with widely fluctuating costs. One useful technique is to partition a center into its principal component parts and to cost each part separately. This modular approach allows the analyst (and the decision maker) to consider a number of possible versions by adding or deleting various modules. An example of such a modular structure is shown in the Appendix.

Cost analysis in support of policy analysis, which is commonly termed systems cost analysis, is different from other types of cost analysis in terms of the following characteristics:[4] end-product orientation, extended time hori-

[4] The characteristics of systems cost analysis discussed herein were drawn from: J. D. Mc-Cullough, *Cost Analysis for Planning-Programming-Budgeting Cost-Benefit Studies,* Santa Monica, Calif., The RAND Corporation, 1966. For additional information on this subject, see particularly: Gene Fisher, In: Novick, *Program Budgeting,* Chap. 3; Quade, *Analysis for Military Decisions;* Charles Hitch and Roland McKean, *The Economics of Defense in the Nuclear Age,* Cambridge, Harvard University Press, 1960; M. V. Jones, *System Cost Analysis: A Management Tool for Decision Making,* Bedford, Mass., The MITRE Corporation, 1964, TM–4063; J. P. Large, ed., *Concepts and Procedures of Cost Analysis,* Santa Monica, Calif., The RAND Corporation, 1963, RM–3589–PR; H. P. Hatry, *The Use of Cost Estimates in Cost-Effectiveness Analysis,* Washington, D.C., Office of Assistant Secretary of Defense (Comptroller) Programming Office, 1965; David Novick, *System and Total Force Cost Analysis,* Santa Monica, Calif., The RAND Corporation, 1961, RM–2695; James G. Abert, "Structuring Cost-Effectiveness Analysis," *Logistics Review and Military Logistics Journal,* 2(7):19–34, July 1966; J. W. Noah, *Concepts and Techniques for Summarizing Defense System Costs,* Washington, D.C., Center for Naval Analysis, 1965; Edward B. Berman, *Cost Analysis in Theory and Practice,* McLean, Va., Research Analysis Corporation, 1964, RAC 161.1. For a bibliography on military systems cost analysis, see P. A. DonVito, *Annotated Bibliography on Systems Cost Analysis,* Santa Monica, Calif., The RAND Corporation, 1966, RM–4848–PR.

zon, incremental costing, life cycle costs, dollars as a measure of resources, and analytical approach and statistical techniques.

END-PRODUCT ORIENTATION

The end-product orientation of cost analysis reflects the requirement—in the general model—that the analysis address the resources necessary to achieve units of output, which, in turn, represent a means for accomplishing defined objectives. The total costs should reflect the total resources used by the system in reaching that objective; that is, the total cost of the decision in terms of dollars and other scarce resources (for example, technical personnel).[5]

Policy analyses often fail to consider the total system cost as it relates to end products. Unfortunately, the analyses succumb to the traditionally narrow definition of "program," which often refers to a proposed expenditure for some purpose which may be, in reality, only a part of the system or subsystem under consideration. For example, costs for a comprehensive health center may (incorrectly) exclude the salaries of personnel paid by a different source.[6]

EXTENDED TIME HORIZON

Cost analysis, as a tool for long-range planning, must take a long view and a wide view. The time horizon must be sufficiently extended to encompass development time, and also must include a sufficiently long period of system operation to account fully for the benefits. Of course, as one proceeds further into the future, the uncertainties become greater. Program costs should be projected for at least five years, although this can be difficult to accomplish. Costs for medical care have risen during the past decade at a rate approximately twice that of the Consumer Price Index (CPI). It is never known at what rate medical care costs will increase in the future.

---

[5] Technically, total costs should be the "opportunity cost" of the decision; that is, the value foregone by not spending the money for the best alternative to the decision. The cost of the program chosen, however, is an adequate approximation for opportunity cost.

[6] Many health delivery programs are funded by several sources. It is important to include *all* costs from *all* sources in the estimates.

If health status for a client group is expected to improve, per capita costs (in terms of constant dollars) could decline. Table 2 shows the estimated effectiveness of a comprehensive health care program serving a low-income community of 25,000 persons. According to these data, these persons should realize substantial reductions in numerous indices. For example, the annual number of days in hospital per 1,000 persons would decline from 1,370 to 960 after five years. Restricted activity days per person per year would decline from 22 to 17.6. This should result in decreased requirements for health services and, therefore, in lower costs.[7]

INCREMENTAL COSTING

Cost analysis in program analysis is an application of the economic concept of marginal analysis. Marginal analysis is different from the accounting concept of associating total costs (including an allocated share of indirect expense) to an end item. The incremental cost of a program is the net difference between its total cost and the cost of an alternative program. In policy analysis, it is the *incremental* cost that is most relevant.

The government is more often a purchaser than a direct provider of services. In some instances (for example, when a hospital provides a service), the cost to the government more closely approximates a fully allocated cost rather than an incremental cost, as the project may be charged for a pro-rata share of the hospital overhead, depreciation of the facilities, teaching, etc. For example, the incremental cost of adding a clinic to an existing hospital should exclude the cost of existing hospital space, depreciation, and other overhead expense, because those costs are already being borne by the hospital. In such instances, the price—from a marginal analysis standpoint—may include sunk (that is, previously spent) costs.[8] This cost to the government, of purchasing services from the private sector, might most accurately be termed a price either established by the state or locale, or by the supplier of the service (for example, the hospital).

---

[7] For example, lowering the hospitalization rate from 1,370 days per 1,000 population to 960 days per 1,000 population (as shown in Table 2) should result in a saving approximating the incremental difference in hospitalization cost for the relevant population.

[8] For example, depreciation charges are sunk costs arising from action taken in the past and unaffected by any subsequent decision.

Table 2.
Comprehensive Health Care Program
Estimated Effects of Program Serving a Low-Income Community of 25,000. Estimated Effectiveness by Year of Operation*

Indices	2nd Year	3rd Year	4th Year	5th Year	Total 5 Years	Baseline Rate Without Program	Estimated Rate After 5 Years
Hospital days saved	0	4,000	7,000	10,500	21,500	1,370 days/1,000	960 days/1,000
Hospital admissions averted	0	200	350	500	1,050	140/1,000	120/1,000
Emergency room visits averted	150	350	500	500	1,500	140/1,000	120/1,000
Disability days averted							
Restricted activity	26,000	50,000	86,000	112,000	274,000	22 days/year	17.6
Bed disability	14,000	37,000	50,000	63,000	164,000	10 days/year	7.5
Work loss	10,000	20,000	30,000	40,000	100,000	8 days/year	6.4
Infant lives saved	2	4.5	7.2	11.5	25.2	41/1,000 LB	25/1,000 LB
Maternal lives saved	.05	.12	.25	.28	.7	.9/1,000 LB	.45/1,000 LB
Cervical cancer in situ detected	1.7	3.0	3.5	3.5	11.7		25% screened/year
Tuberculosis							
Deaths averted	.14	.27	.46	.57	1.44	9.8/100,000	7.3/100,000
Cases averted	0	2.6	4.2	4.8	11.6	74.9/100,000	56/100,000
Influ-pneu. deaths averted	1.3	2.8	4.2	5.5	13.8	55.4/100,000	33.5/100,000
Children with checkups							
% under age 6	35%	50%	60%	60%		25%	60%
% age 6–16	20%	25%	33%	33%		15%	33%
Dental visits/person/year						.85/per/yr.	1.5/per/yr.
Prenatal care 1st trimester	10%	20%	35%	40%		10%	40%
% not immunized							
DPT (age 1–4)	20%	15%	12%	10%		22.5%	10%
Polio (age 1–4)	18%	15%	10%	7.5%		20%	7.5%

* Assumes no change in indices first year of operation.
Source: Department of Health, Education, and Welfare, *Delivery of Health Services for the Poor.* Washington, D.C., December 1967.

Figure 5 illustrates the costs of two alternative delivery vehicles considered in *Delivery of Health Services for the Poor.* Illustration I depicts the comparative costs of the Comprehensive Health Center (CHC) and Improved Outpatient Department (OPD) as presented in the analysis (we have adjusted them somewhat for the purpose of comparability). According to the analysis, no CHC existed. An OPD did exist, which cost $50 per capita for delivery of outpatient services to 25,000 poor persons. Therefore, according to the usual concepts of systems cost analysis, the marginal costs are $110 for the CHC and $42 ($92 —$50) for the OPD. The remaining portion of the $92 total cost for the OPD ($50) is represented by the existing system. This, however, is an incorrect assumption for the OPD. Actually, $92 represents the true *total annual operating cost to the public sector*; thus, in comparing costs of alternatives, the total annual costs for the delivery vehicle are relevant, as shown in illustration II. If only the $42 increment were considered the total annual cost, the cost of operating the OPD would be understated. In developing costs for a program to improve OPD's, however, the marginal costs constitute the *new additional funds* that should be programmed (assuming the existing programs are to be continued).

Illustrations III and IV in Figure 5 depict additional perturbations in the consideration of costs. Illustration III shows the actual federal share of the operating costs due to different fund-matching requirements. Thus, while the Federal Government, through the Office of Economic Opportunity, provides 90 percent of the CHC funds, it also provides the $42 increment for improving the OPD and approximately 50 percent of the remaining $50 through other programs (for example, Medicaid). Illustration IV shows the type of phenomenon discussed earlier; that is, when a hospital charges a price for operating a delivery vehicle that exceeds the incremental cost, the difference may be allocated costs. Thus, the assumption that incremental costs of the improvements in a system correspond to costs to the government might not be absolutely correct in practice. This might, in fact, result in the CHC becoming the preferred alternative from a cost standpoint.

The impact of alternative funding mechanisms on the selection of alternatives also must be considered. This is highly relevant in that it not only influences the cost to the Federal Government but the cost to the state or local government as well (which often decides which programs to pursue). An example of the impact of financing mechanisms may be seen in Table 3. These data, developed by the author in an analysis of maternal and child health programs in a city, show the comparative costs of providing maternity

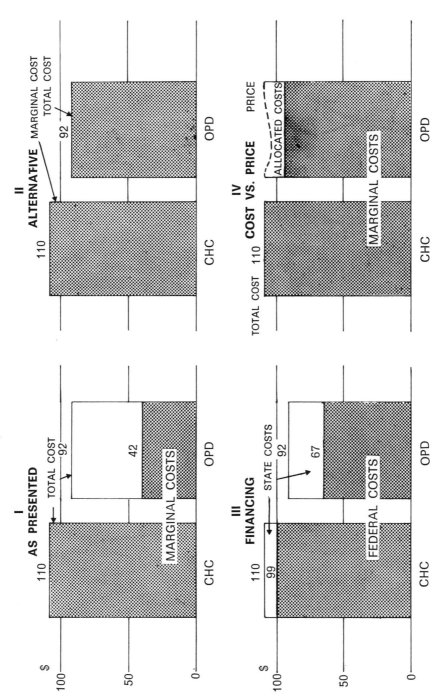

Figure 5. Annual per capita cost for delivering outpatient services to 25,000 poor persons.

Table 3.

Total Costs of Alternative Delivery Vehicles
Providing Maternity Care—Cost Per Patient

	Maternal and Infant Care Project		Neighborhood Health Center		Private MD	
	$	%	$	%	$	%
Total Cost	313	100	199	100	175	100
Federal Share	282	90	103	51.7	90	51.7
State Share	31	10	96	48.3	85	48.3

care through alternative delivery vehicles—Maternal and Infant Care Project, Neighborhood Health Center, and Private MD (for outpatient care only). Although, from an analytical standpoint, the total cost of the decision is the relevant one (resulting in the selection of the Private MD or perhaps the Neighborhood Health Center),[9] the rational decision maker at the state level would be inclined to pursue the least efficient alternative (Maternal and Infant Care Project), as the cost to the state is lower than in the more efficient alternatives. Conversely, the Federal Government could favor one of the other alternatives (probably the private MD), assuming effectiveness is equal for all three alternatives.

LIFE CYCLE COSTS

Cost categories (research and development, investment, and operating) are intended to encompass the costs of a program from conception to phase-out. Their phasing is illustrated in Figure 6. Research and development costs are attributable to development decisions, and the choice is made from among feasible alternatives at that stage. Investment costs normally represent

---

[9] A major factor in the decision could be that Private MD's ·are unwilling to practice in poverty areas, but Neighborhood Health Centers might have less difficulty in attracting them.

one-time costs for fixed assets such as facilities and major equipment. Operating costs are related to the manner and length of time that the system should be operating. These costs cover the day-to-day operation of the system and include such major expenses as personnel salaries and benefits, supplies, rentals, and maintenance.

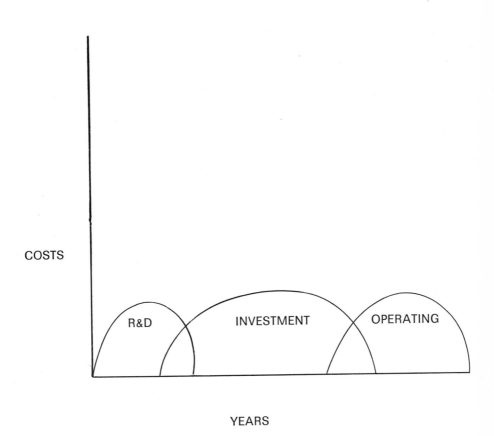

Figure 6. Cost categories illustrated.

DOLLARS AS A MEASURE OF RESOURCES

The total systems cost cannot be determined solely by adding the dollar costs of such items as equipment, personnel, facilities, and supplies. Whenever possible, dollars are the measure of the value of resources required; but certain resources are scarce and should be expressed in terms of their physical quantity. In health policy analysis, scarce critical resources such as professional manpower (for example, physicians and nurses) should be given separate attention in the analysis.

The question of the extent to which dollars are an adequate measure of resources or inputs must be resolved from the viewpoint of whether they can *readily* purchase other inputs. It is not difficult to purchase such things as desks, most equipment, and office supplies; although, we who have been disturbed over the slowness of suppliers in meeting delivery schedules could argue the point. Because in most areas of the United States there appears to be a far greater demand for than supply of physicians and nurses, they are considered scarce resources. Even if dollars are available to pay them, a program probably will have difficulty hiring physicians and nurses. This problem is particularly acute in central city and rural areas. For this reason, "dollars" is not an adequate proxy for physicians and nurses; their availability also must be considered. Thus, the question of the extent to which the availability of these personnel acts as a constraint to the feasibility of the alternatives should be explicitly addressed. An important part of the analysis could be determining how the scarce manpower is to be obtained.

ANALYTICAL APPROACH AND STATISTICAL TECHNIQUES

Statistical techniques can be used to determine Cost Estimating Relationships (CER's) suitable for projecting costs of future systems. Scatter diagrams, regression analysis, and correlation analysis are examples of the techniques used to develop CER's. For example, there tends to be a linear relationship between operating costs of both inpatient and outpatient health services and the number of patients receiving these services. Figure 7 illustrates such a relationship. In this example, total operating costs for similar health clinics providing services to various numbers of patients are plotted on a scatter diagram. Predictably, total operating costs increase as the number of patients served increases. Assuming that the services to be offered by a new clinic

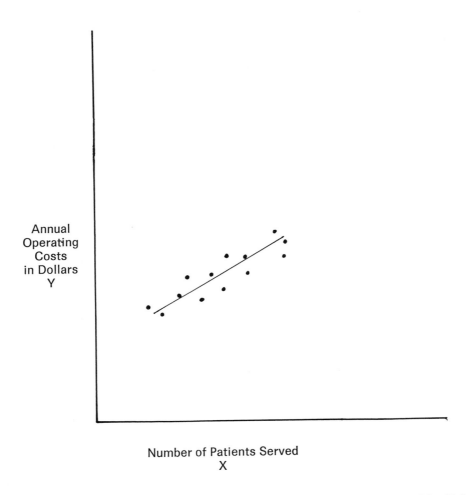

Figure 7. Operating costs and patients served by comprehensive health clinics.

and the type of patients to be served are comparable to those represented on the scatter diagram, the annual operating costs may be found by determining the number of patients to be served. The relationship between operating costs (Y) and number of patients served (X) may be crudely determined by drawing a straight line roughly equidistant between the points on the scatter diagram.[10]

A more refined technique also can be employed, using standard mathematical procedures of linear regression analysis. Here, the formula $Y = a + bX$ is used to determine the line of "best fit," based on statistical estimates of the values of a and b. Where more than one explanatory variable (X) is used, multiple rather than simple regression analysis may be employed. The resulting equations are termed Cost Estimating Relationships (CER's).[11]

Measuring Program Effectiveness

Having analyzed the input side of a model, we will now approach the output side. The difficulties encountered in using a composite index of health, and the shortcomings that result from using only measures of morbidity and mortality, were discussed previously in this chapter. In this section, we will concentrate on developing measures of system effectiveness that will assist the decision maker in making more informed, rational program decisions.[12] We will consider methods for measuring effectiveness that are capable of being implemented, given the current state-of-the-art and availability of data.

Alternative approaches for measuring effectiveness may be expressed as follows:

1. Derive a cardinal utility function, such that a numerical value is assigned to Φ for alternative effectiveness vectors.[13]

---

[10] Of course, while the line can reasonably represent the relationship between operating costs and patients served, this is true only within the range of the observed data points. Extrapolation beyond this range can be misleading and should be avoided.

[11] Regression analysis is explained in most intermediate statistics tests; for example, see Edward C. Bryant, *Statistical Analysis*, New York, McGraw-Hill, 1966.

[12] This discussion excludes the question of political rationality. It is assumed, however, that political implications are considered at a subsequent stage.

[13] Where effectiveness vectors are $X_1, X_2, \ldots, X_n$ and $\Phi = \Phi (X_1, X_2, \ldots X_n)$. See John von Neuman and O. Morgenstern, *Theory of Games and Economic Behavior*, Princeton, N.J., Princeton University Press, 1944; Peter C. Fishburn, *Decision and Value Theory*, New York, Wiley, 1964; H. Chernoff and L. E. Moses, *Elementary Decision Theory*, New York, Wiley, 1957; and A. H. Packer, "Applying Cost-Effectiveness Concepts," p. 238.

2. Using ordinal utility theory, do not assume that numerical values can be assigned to each effectiveness vector, but that they can be ordered (one vector is better, worse, or equal to another).[14]
3. Present the complete effectiveness vectors corresponding to the alternative system configurations to the decision maker, who then makes his own choice.

The choice among the three alternative approaches suggested above will be largely determined by the quality of the data available and the precision required to choose among alternative programs. It cannot be emphasized too strongly that, in medical program analysis, the prime concern is with decision making under conditions of extreme uncertainty—particularly in estimating program effectiveness. Uncertainty is the rule, rather than the exception, and its existence is a relative phenomenon that, in most instances, will be present to some degree. What we are seeking in this discussion is a satisfactory way to deal with this uncertainty.

Figure 8 presents an illustrative, hypothetical cost-effectiveness graph with three cost-effectiveness surfaces (the cross-hatched regions A, B, C). Each surface has one cost-effectiveness point (a,b,c) representing the expected cost-effectiveness values. Each of the latter three represents the cost-effectiveness estimated for an alternative program.

The first approach described above would require placing a numerical scale on the horizontal axis or abscissa of the cost-effectiveness graph. In the second approach, the scale of the abscissa becomes indeterminate, and relative—but not absolute—effectiveness can be determined. For example, point c is more effective than point b, and point b is more effective than point a. There is no way to measure the quantity of difference, however, and the decision as to whether the additional effectiveness is worth the added cost is a matter of value judgments held by the analyst, expert opinion, and the decision maker. In the third approach, separate graphs may be constructed for each element of the effectiveness vector (that is, each evaluation criterion) and presented to the decision maker.

[14] The ordinal rankings may be expressed in subscript convention as:
$$V_1 \geq V_2 \geq \ldots \geq V_j \ldots \geq V_k \geq K_r.$$

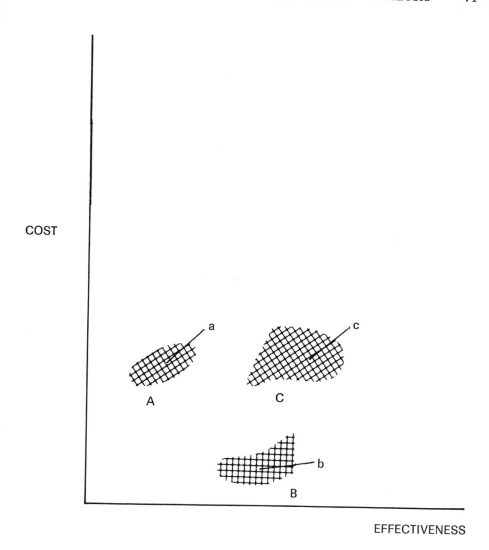

Figure 8. Cost-effectiveness alternatives with uncertainty.

A. H. Packer, who suggested the three alternative approaches, states:

> The three alternative approaches are not mutually exclusive. A numerical-valued (cardinal) utility function can be both a useful conceptual device and a goal to be sought even if it cannot be achieved in an operational sense. Using this approach, an attempt can be made to combine as many elements as possible in an effectiveness vector. That is, if a number (say, m) of utility functions can be defined by combining sets of the n variables, then the policymaker can be presented with a shorter and more meaningful effectiveness vector of the form $\Phi = \Phi_1, \Phi_2, \ldots, \Phi_m$ where m is less than n. He must then reconcile these effectiveness measures. Analogies can be observed in industrial situations. Ideally, the basic objective may be to maximize the vaguely defined "long run profit"; in fact, the policy maker must reconcile an effectiveness written in terms of current profit, market share, liquidity, public image, etc.[15]

In view of the conceptual and analytical difficulties involved in determining a composite index of health, we must reluctantly reject—for the present—the first alternative approach for measuring effectiveness. This is not to suggest that research should not continue, with the hope that the serious problems will be surmounted. What it does suggest is that the use of such composite measures is analytically not desirable, in view of the great complexity and multidimensional nature of health program objectives and the lack of data.

A major shortcoming of benefit-cost analysis, a form of cardinal utility, is that it quantifies economic benefits only and places greater value upon programs aimed at persons who are in or about to enter their most productive years. Benefits to very young children and older persons are comparatively low, because the former group will not earn income until so far into the future that the discount rate greatly reduces the present value, and the latter group has only limited productive years of life remaining so future income is low. For example, at a low (3 percent) discount rate, the value to society of a male 1 to 5 years old is $100,000; 25 to 35 years old, $150,000; and 65 to 70 years old, $25,000.[16]

Combinations of the second and third alternative approaches should be used, and these will be illustrated later in this chapter.

---

[15] A. H. Packer, "Applying Cost-Effectiveness Concepts," p. 238.
[16] U.S. Department of Health, Education, and Welfare. *Motor Vehicle Accident Prevention Program.* Washington, D.C., U.S. Government Printing Office, 1966. p. 70.

Discounting

Discounting is most relevant to a cost-benefit analysis in which future benefit streams, expressed in terms of dollars, may be sensitive to the discount rate. It is considerably less important to program analyses in which benefits are not expressed in dollar terms; thus, only program costs could be discounted. Where costs vary significantly between alternatives over a period of years, discounting should be used.

Because cost-benefit analysis is, in itself, inadequate for presenting the decision maker with criteria for choice, discounting is of relatively little concern in health program analysis. The relative ranking of programs normally will not change if program costs only are discounted. In cases where cost-benefit analysis is deemed appropriate (this should be in conjunction with other techniques), one or more discount rates should be employed.[17]

Selecting the Preferred Alternatives

Thus far in the analytical process, we have considered the steps leading to the determination of the preferred alternatives. At this point, the analyst should have identified the costs and effectiveness (to the extent possible) of each alternative under consideration in his model. Unfortunately, analyses tend to break down at this point, and the decision maker frequently is left with unrelated costs and effectiveness measures. The correct criteria for selection are the comparative costs *and* effectiveness considered together.

ALTERNATIVE DISEASE CONTROL PROGRAMS

Packer suggests a technique that describes disability states in terms of case-months, and seeks a state in which:

> Any possible alternative to the (optimal) decision will create additional case-months in some disability state without any offsetting reductions in some other state. If it can be assumed that the disability states can be strictly ordered (e.g.,

---

[17] Alternative rates of (say) 5, 10, and 15 percent could be considered. The lowest rate should be the rate paid by the Federal Government on long-term loans; the highest rate might approximate the opportunity cost of the proposed expenditure. For a discussion of the major issues involved, see Robert L. Banks and Arnold Kotz, "The Program Budget and the Interest Rate for Public Investment," *Public Administration Review,* 26(4):283–292, December 1966.

limited mobility is strictly preferred to confinement), the area of unambiguous choice can be further extended. In this instance any possible alternative to the "optimal" decision will create additional case-months in some less preferred state at least equal to the offsetting number of cases in the more preferred state.

These concepts may be illustrated by a simple example. Assume that five alternative disease control programs (A, B, C, D, E) are available and that the estimated case-months in each disability state associated with each are as given in [Table 4].

As a first guess, assume that Program C is the optimum program. Program C is unambiguously superior to A . . . for each disability state the number of case-months associated with Program A equals or exceeds that for C. Program C is unambiguously superior to B by the second criterion. The relative reduction in the number of case-months in (the more preferred) state 4 associated with Program B is at least offset by the increase in case-months in (the less preferred) state 5. A comparison between Programs C and D is only a more complicated case of that between Programs C and B. Again C is unambiguously superior, since reductions in case-months in more preferred states are at least offset by increases in case-months in the less preferred states. A comparison between Programs C and E illustrates the point previously made that no general solution can be found. The relative evaluation of 1,000 case-months of restricted activity against one additional month of premature death is ultimately a subjective judgment.[18]

Table 4.
Estimated Case-Months Resulting from
Five Alternative Programs

Disability State	*Disease Control Programs*				
	A	*B*	*C*	*D*	*E*
1. Minor Disability	1,000	1,000	1,000	900	1,000
2. Restricted Disability	1,100	1,000	1,000	1,100	0
3. Limited Activity	1,200	1,000	1,000	900	1,000
4. Limited Mobility	1,000	900	1,000	900	1,000
5. Confined	1,000	1,100	1,000	900	1,000
6. Death	1,000	1,000	1,000	1,300	1,001

Source: A. H. Packer, "Applying Cost-Effectiveness Concepts," p. 241.

[18] A. H. Packer, "Applying Cost-Effectiveness Concepts," pp. 240–241. While benefit-cost analysis with its single measure of cardinal utility is conceptually superior to Packer's multidimensional approach, Packer's technique actually better represents the decision maker's criteria of relative preference. The apparently unambiguous benefit-cost ratio is illusory, and a multidimensional presentation is superior.

This approach is feasible and, in fact, similar data are required in order to compute benefits. This should be done in conjunction with the computation of benefit-cost ratios, and the decision maker should be presented with complete effectiveness vectors and related costs.

ALTERNATIVE HEALTH SERVICES PROGRAMS[19]

The next problem to consider is how to use cost-effectiveness criteria to choose among health service alternatives in which multiple effectiveness measures are determined. The basic analytical problem is that the costs cover the entire program (or major portions thereof) under consideration and, with few exceptions, cannot be partitioned into parts solely attributable unambiguously to only one effectiveness indicator. This presents a classic, joint-cost/joint-product problem in which there is no satisfactory best way to allocate costs and effectiveness. It was previously noted that attempts to establish a composite index of health have not been successful and that benefit-cost analysis in itself is inadequate as a basis for decision. Both of these collapse effectiveness into one measure to allow for the attribution of cost inputs to comparable outputs. Since we cannot accomplish this, given the current state-of-the-analytical-art, a less conceptually satisfying, yet more workable alternative, must be pursued.

In this illustrative case, the analytical question is: Which alternative delivery vehicles should be selected to provide outpatient medical services to the poor? For two of the alternatives—Comprehensive Health Center and Improved Outpatient Clinic—12 effectiveness measures are derived, and quantities are estimated. For the remainder of the alternatives—Comprehensive Group Practice, Group Practice, and Solo Practice—effectiveness is not estimated.

---

[19] Before proceeding further, a note of caution is required. This section frequently will compare comprehensive programs with noncomprehensive alternatives that do not address as wide a range of health problems. One may only estimate effectiveness in a few of the most severe categories (for example, infant mortality). Thus the comparisons are not truly consistent. Alternatively, one could assume that a comprehensive program includes all that the potential categorical programs include. Then one should sum all categorical programs applicable to such a population and compare the total costs and effectiveness with the comprehensive program, or, perhaps alternatively, assume effectiveness to be equal for both and compare the costs. No precise adjustment for this problem is offered in the ensuing discussion, as such data are not now available. The data presented in the analysis will be used to illustrate a methodology, but the reader is urged to bear in mind that the effectiveness of the comprehensive alternatives is incompletely stated and that the categorical alternatives are not completely comparable to them.

Table 5 depicts the comparative effectiveness and resource requirements of the two alternatives for which effectiveness was computed. Strictly from the standpoint of effectiveness, the Comprehensive Health Center is clearly dominant, as it either equals or exceeds the Improved Outpatient Clinic in all the effectiveness categories. Two alternatives are shown under program costs for the Improved Outpatient Clinic (namely, $5.1 and $12.4 million) for the two ways of expressing the marginal costs that were discussed earlier.[20] Clearly, in each case, the Improved Outpatient Clinic is cheaper than the Comprehensive Health Center. Due to the joint-cost/joint-product problem previously described, there is no rigorously acceptable way to choose between the two alternatives. In view of the incremental effectiveness ob-

Table 5.

Estimated 5-Year Effectiveness and Costs of Alternatives
Serving a Low-Income Community of 25,000 Persons

Effectiveness Categories	*Out-patient Clinic (1)*	*Comprehensive Health Center (2)*	*Difference*	
			Actual	*%*
Hospital days saved	21,500	21,500	0	0
Hospital admissions averted	1,050	1,050	0	0
Emergency room visits averted	950	1,500	550	58
Restricted activity days averted	188,000	274,000	86,000	46
Bed disability days averted	118,000	164,000	46,000	39
Work loss days averted	65,000	100,000	35,000	54
Infant lives saved	14.7	25.2	10.5	71
Maternal lives saved	.54	.7	.16	30
Cervical cancer in situ detected	9.1	11.7	2.6	29
Tuberculosis deaths averted	.74	1.44	.7	95
Tuberculosis cases averted	5.2	11.6	6.4	123
Influenza-pneumonia deaths averted	6.9	13.8	6.9	100
Program Costs ($000)				
Alternative 1	5,130	14,600	9,470	184
Alternative 2	12,350	14,600	2,250	18
MD's required	25	25	0	0

[20] We concluded that the correct way was Alternative 2, which represents the marginal cost to *both* the Federal Government and other sources. Alternative 1 represents only the cost to the Federal Government for the grants proposed, although Figure 5 demonstrated that the true cost to the Federal Government is understated.

tained from the incremental difference in costs between the two programs, however, the Comprehensive Health Center probably is the more attractive. This is because the increase of 18 percent in expenditures results in significantly larger percentage increments in effectiveness, with the exception of the categories "hospital days saved" and "hospital admissions averted." As these categories are redundant, they may be collapsed into one category— hospital days saved, for which the difference is 0. The decision as to which is the preferred alternative ultimately depends upon the decision maker's relative preference for hospital days saved in comparison to the other effectiveness categories.[21] Obviously, if Alternative 1 ($5.1 million) were accepted as the correct marginal cost, the Outpatient Clinic would be a considerably more attractive alternative.

No effectiveness measures (except number of patients treated) are estimated for the other alternative delivery vehicles. For this situation, ordinal preference might be obtained by calling on expert medical opinion as the criterion. Expert medical opinion indicates that this results in the following ordinal scale:

Ordinal Rank	*Delivery Vehicle*
1	Comprehensive Health Center
2	Comprehensive Group Practice
3	Group Practice
4	Outpatient Clinic
5	Solo Practice

Thus, the preceding example clearly indicates that Comprehensive Group Practice and Group Practice fall (in terms of effectiveness) somewhere between the Comprehensive Health Center and the Outpatient Clinic, while the effectiveness of Solo Practice is below that of the Outpatient Clinic.

The comparative costs of medical services for each of the above is indicated in Table 6. Whether the incremental differences in costs among alternatives are worth the incremental effectiveness becomes the analytical question at this point. Although the Comprehensive Health Center is preferable to the Outpatient Clinic, and the ordinal rankings of all the alternatives

---

[21] These are, of course, cost-effectiveness criteria only. Consideration also should be given to the uncertainties in the effectiveness estimates, as well as to institutional factors—for example, that the Outpatient Clinics are already in existence and require only marginal improvements while the Comprehensive Health Centers normally would be completely new with all the attendant problems of sponsorship, start-up time, etc.

Table 6.

Five-Year Medical Service Resource Requirements of
Alternative Delivery Vehicles Serving 25,000 Persons

Resources	Compre-hensive Health Center	Compre-hensive Group Practice	Group Practice	Improved Out-patient Clinic	Solo Practice
COSTS ($ million)	9.3	7.1	6.9	7.9	6.9
Critical Manpower MD's RN's	25 12	26 12	24 12	25 12	29 9

are known, there is no precise way of choosing among them based on clear, cost-effectiveness criteria. The selection must, therefore, be a matter of judgment.

Implementation

The work of the analyst is not quite finished. He must prepare a report, carefully documenting such things as his analysis procedure, data, and assumptions. He should include considerations of alternative financing mechanisms and sources of funds and should be prepared to submit an implementation plan. The results of the analysis must be sold to the decision maker and to those persons who influence him. Institutional, bureaucratic, and political factors must be addressed if the results are to be implemented. All of these things could well be the subject of a separate monograph.

Evaluating and Monitoring

Policy analysis begins a management cycle which should be essentially circular, as illustrated in Figure 9. Policy analysis and planning must be followed by implementation of the alternatives selected by the decision maker. Data collection and reporting procedures should be established so that reports on program operations are routinely generated.

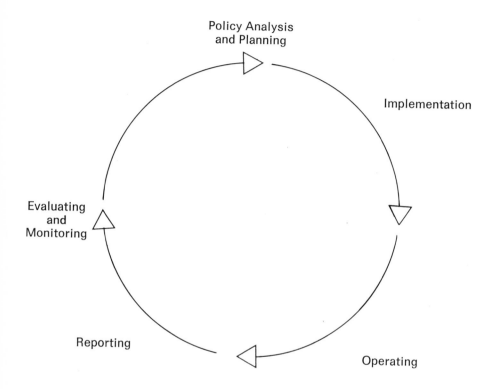

Figure 9. The management cycle.

Evaluation and monitoring are facilitated considerably where reporting systems are established. Reporting may be primarily on operating data. In order to facilitate evaluation, data must be collected consistent with the measure of effectiveness used in the policy analysis. Later, this simplifies analyzing the cost-effectiveness of the programs in light of the objectives and evaluation criteria previously established. Chapter 6 presents a specific evaluation case history.

Part II

Case Histories

INTRODUCTION

Three cases, each illustrating a different type of policy analysis, are discussed in Part II: Maternal and Child Health Care Programs (Chapter 4), Simulation and Cost-Effectiveness Analysis of New York's Emergency Ambulance Service (Chapter 5), and Evaluation of a Family Planning Program for American Indians (Chapter 6).

The Maternal and Child Health Care Program is a "classical" type of policy analysis, proceeding in a series of steps conforming somewhat to those discussed in Part I of this book. It is an excellent example of how an analyst may begin with an extremely broad policy problem, reduce it to parts that are manageable analytically, make good use of admittedly inadequate available data, and present reasonably clear policy alternatives for consideration. This analysis had a significant impact on the policy process in the U.S. Department of Health, Education, and Welfare.

In contrast, the Simulation and Cost-Effectiveness Analysis of New York's Emergency Ambulance Service addressed a considerably more narrow issue. The essential analytical steps that were followed, however, are quite similar to those used in the first case and suggested in Part I of this book. Because the issue was rather narrowly circumscribed, used relatively "hard" data, and dealt with the spatial allocation of ambulances, an operations research tool—in this case simulation—was used. This case also had a significant impact on the policy-making process, and a substantial reallocation of the New York City ambulance fleet resulted.

The third case differs from the preceding two, first, because it is an evaluation as opposed to a policy analysis per se. It is essentially a retrospective look at the effectiveness of a family planning program for American Indians. The procedures followed in this retrospective evaluation, however, are quite similar to those that should be used in conducting a policy analysis. In fact, an integral part of any policy analysis is the evaluation of the major alternatives under consideration. Thus, this evaluation follows a similar procedure up to the point where the cost and effectiveness of the existing programs are estimated. It does not, however, take the further steps of considering alternatives to existing programs and attempting to evaluate them in terms of similar cost and effectiveness measures.

The foregoing cases may be considered "successes" in terms of the most important criterion used in evaluating the effectiveness of policy analysis itself—their impact on the policy-making process.

Several conclusions emerged from the maternal and child health care analysis. Two of these conclusions resulted in new legislation being requested from Congress. Clearly, a program of early case-finding and treatment of handicapping conditions was called for. It also was apparent that a large number of children did not have access to good medical care and could not be provided with conventional pediatric services due to an acute shortage of doctors. Means had to be found to use medical manpower more efficiently. The Social Security Amendments of 1967 included provisions for programs of early case-finding and treatment of defects and chronic handicapping conditions in children, and for research and demonstration programs in the training and use of physician assistants.

The emergency ambulance service analysis resulted in a significant redeployment of ambulances in the city of New York. Initially, a major conclusion was that one satellite station should be established. Carrying the analysis to its logical conclusion, however, required more complete decentralization of ambulances to curbside locations; this was finally implemented. The enthusiastic response of Mayor Lindsey and the apparently successful new system for emergency ambulance service caused the Department of Housing and Urban Development to package the system for implementation in other cities as well as in New York.

The evaluation of family planning programs for American Indians demonstrated the continued efficacy of providing such programs. The programs have continued to expand and, indeed, now represent one of the highest priority programs offered by the Indian Health Service. In this case, the evaluation served to confirm a previously determined course of action and provided impetus for continued expansion of that program.

CHAPTER 4

MATERNAL AND CHILD HEALTH CARE PROGRAMS[1]

The Secretary of the U.S. Department of Health, Education, and Welfare was faced with the problem of deciding which programs should be pursued to improve the health status of mothers and children in the United States. A policy analysis was conducted that proposed specific objectives and reviewed national needs for maternal and child health, described major ongoing maternal and child health care programs, and estimated the costs and effects of programs designed to meet the proposed objectives. Primarily, the analysis addressed the need for, the costs, and the effects of medical care for children in low-income families. It did not address important related questions regarding the effects on child health exerted by changes in income level, environmental health programs, improved nutrition, communicable disease control, or accident prevention programs; nor did it address the problems of the unequal geographical distribution of physicians, the need for strengthening obstetric and pediatric departments, or the status of state laws governing the medical and nursing practices.

The analysis proposed the following specific objectives for the health of children living in poverty: reduction of infant mortality; prevention, correction, or amelioration of chronic handicapping conditions; and reduction of unmet dental needs. Major ongoing child health care programs, program costs, numbers of children reached, and inadequacies in present programs were discussed. The bulk of the analysis estimated total cost, manpower requirements, and effects of the following alternatives:

1. Comprehensive maternal and child health care programs.
2. Programs to provide early case-finding and treatment of congenital and other chronic disorders.

---

[1] This information was obtained from: U.S. Department of Health, Education, and Welfare, *Maternal and Child Health Care Programs*, Washington, D.C., U.S. Government Printing Office, 1967.

3. A program to provide early case-finding of vision and hearing defects.
4. Programs to reduce unmet dental needs.
5. Intensive care units for high-risk premature and other infants.
6. A program of support for expanded family planning services.

The costs, manpower requirements, and estimated effects of these programs in a low-income urban or rural community of 50,000 people were estimated, and the cost-effectiveness of these programs was compared in accomplishing each of the child health objectives.

Objectives, National Needs, and Evaluation Criteria

Although all of the objectives relate to the health of the child population in general, the analysis gives priority to accomplishing the objectives for children in the most disadvantaged areas—characterized as health-depressed areas. Health-depressed areas can best be defined in terms of the infant mortality rate, the proportion of families living in poverty, and the proportion of substandard housing. Simply stated, the analysis defines a health-depressed area as an area in which the infant mortality rate is high, because infant mortality has long been used as the best single indicator of the health status of a community. Generally, infant mortality rates are highest in areas characterized by low-income persons in poor housing areas. In urban areas, health-depressed areas can be defined as census tracts or combinations of census tracts; in rural areas, health-depressed areas can be defined as counties or combinations of adjoining counties with high infant mortality rates.

OBJECTIVES

Following are definitions of some objectives:

1. Make needed maternal and child health care services available and accessible to all; in particular, to all expectant mothers and children in health-depressed areas. It was recognized that there is no universal index of good or bad health among children. In order to obtain an operationally usable measure of health status, it was decided to focus

principally upon the health problems which are highly prevalent, highly adverse, and which can be mitigated—and even avoided— given proper health care: infant mortality, chronic handicapping conditions, and bad teeth. It was expected that health care directed toward these problems would also yield important benefits to the general health of the mothers and their children.

Progress toward the major objective was to be measured, at least to some extent, by progress toward accomplishing each of the following subordinate objectives.

2. Reduce infant mortality rates, particularly in health-depressed areas.
3. Reduce the number of chronic handicapping conditions, the incidence of preventable handicapping conditions, and the prevalence of uncorrected handicapping conditions. In particular, reduce congenital defects; mental retardation; vision, hearing, and speech defects; and mental and emotional disorders.
4. Reduce unmet dental needs, particularly in health-depressed areas.

National Child Health Needs[2]

The analysis described major ongoing child health care programs; federal, state, and local costs of those programs for fiscal years 1965, 1966, and 1967 (as available); and numbers of children reached. It concluded that present programs fall short of providing adequate health care for all mothers and children living in poverty; that the majority of low-income mothers fail to receive adequate maternity care; and that most children of low-income families are deprived of adequate preventive or remedial health care (even after handicapping conditions have been identified in screening programs). It was estimated that, at the present time, at least 800,000 mothers living in poverty require comprehensive prenatal services, but only about a third of a million receive care in maternity clinics under the Maternal and Child Health Care Programs. While some 4 to 5 million children under five years of age are in the poverty group requiring care, only about 1.5 million are receiving such care under the Maternal and Child Health Care Program well-child conferences.

---

[2] This section presents the definition of the problem essentially as it appeared in the report.

MORTALITY

In the United States, the infant mortality rate dropped from 69 deaths per 1,000 live births in 1925–1929, to 47 per 1,000 in 1940, and 26.4 per 1,000 in 1955. This improvement was due chiefly to a reduction in mortality from infectious diseases. In the past decade, there has been little change in infant mortality in this country.

Meanwhile, infant mortality rates in other countries have continued to decline: in 1964, the United States had an infant mortality rate of 24.8 (almost 100,000 infant deaths among slightly over 4,000,000 live births); Sweden ranked first, with an infant mortality rate of 14.2.[3] Assuming the same U.S. birth rate, if the Swedish infant mortality rate had applied in the United States, 42,600 fewer infants would have died in the United States; if the British rate of 20.6 had applied, 16,800 fewer infants would have died.

The existence of wide disparities among infant mortality rates within the United States is another indicator that many infants are dying needlessly. In 1964, state rates ranged from 19.8 in Massachusetts to 39.4 in Mississippi; in the nation as a whole, the rate was 21.6 for white infants and 41.1 for nonwhite infants (see Table 7). Rates for the nation's 3,130 counties vary even more, and rates within counties vary even further. Rates for white and nonwhite infants born in the larger cities generally are similar to those for the country as a whole.

Table 7.
Infant Mortality in the United States, 1964

	Number of Deaths	*Rate Per 1,000 Live Births*
Infant (under 1 year)	99,783	24.8
White	72,728	21.6
Nonwhite	27,055	41.1
Neonatal (under 28 days)	72,026	17.9
White	54,593	16.2
Nonwhite	17,433	26.5
Postneonatal (1 to 11 months)	27,757	6.9
White	18,135	5.4
Nonwhite	9,622	14.6

3 Although slight differences have been noted in the divisions among stillbirths and infant deaths in the United States and in other countries, these differences would only account for approximately 1 death per 1,000 live births.

Higher infant mortality, as well as higher prematurity rates and higher incidence of mental retardation, result from lack of adequate maternity care. Less than 50 percent of low-income women receive care in maternity clinics. In fact, in most of the major cities, one-third to one-half of the women delivered at city hospitals had *no* prenatal care. One-fourth of the excess deaths (and one-fifth of the births) occurred in only 21 of the nation's 3,130 counties (see Table 8).

The data on deaths of children over age one also reveal large disparities between the white and the nonwhite population and among the states, but the numbers of deaths are much smaller.

Table 8.

Counties With At Least 800 Excess Infant Deaths, 1956–1960

Major City	County	County Infant Mortality Rate
Atlanta	Fulton	31.6
Baltimore		33.8
Birmingham	Jefferson	30.1
Chicago	Cook	26.2
Cleveland	Cuyahoga	27.3
Dallas	Dallas	26.3
Detroit	Wayne	26.5
Houston	Harris	28.2
Indianapolis	Marion	27.4
Los Angeles	Los Angeles	24.6
Memphis	Shelby	30.7
Miami	Dade	29.3
Milwaukee	Milwaukee	24.5
Newark	Essex	29.9
New Orleans	New Orleans	33.9
New York		26.0
Philadelphia		32.0
Pittsburgh	Allegheny	23.5
San Antonio	Bexar	31.7
St. Louis		30.3
Washington, D.C.		36.1

CHRONIC CONDITIONS

Chronic conditions include orthopedic, cardiovascular, genitourinary, neurological, mental and emotional, hearing, vision, speech, nutritional, and skin disorders, as well as allergies and nonacute respiratory conditions. Except for data from studies of congenital malformations, little hard data exist on the incidence and prevalence of chronic conditions in children. Populations examined (and conditions counted) in the major studies usually are not comparable. Neither are definitive data available on the extent of disability caused by chronic illness. The following estimates are based on the major studies undertaken over the past decade.

In 1964, Crippled Children's Programs served one-half of one percent of the population under 21 (420,000 children), but the Children's Bureau estimated that more than twice as many needed help under that program.

Tables 9 to 11 give some estimates of the proportions of children with chronic handicapping conditions. In addition, based on a survey of the pertinent literature, Table 11 presents some rough estimates of the proportions of the major handicapping conditions in each diagnostic category that could be prevented or corrected by child health care: approximately 62 percent of these handicapping conditions could be prevented or corrected by comprehensive care up to age 18; approximately 33 percent could be prevented or corrected by case-finding and treatment at appropriate ages in early childhood.

It is estimated that approximately 23 percent of school children require eye care (mainly glasses), but that only approximately 17 percent wear glasses; hence, approximately 3 million more school children ought to have glasses. Amblyopia (blindness in one eye) now occurs in 2 to 3 percent of the population (estimates actually range from 0.5 to 3 percent), although almost all of it is preventable with proper treatment at about age three.

UNMET DENTAL NEEDS

By age five or six, almost all children (97 percent) require some dental care. By age 13, the average child has 11 to 12 decayed, missing, or filled teeth. Almost all children require some dental care each year (to clean and fill teeth and to receive necessary care for gums). The percentages presented in Table 12, therefore, represent conservative estimates of the numbers of

Table 9.

Approximate Proportions of Children With Chronic Conditions
(Both Treated and Untreated)

Conditions	*0*	*3*	*5–6*	*8–9*
			Ages	
Congenital Malformations[a]	7%	6.6%	6.6%	6.6%
Vision Problems		3	8	11
Hearing Problems		1.5	3	4
Psychiatric Problems			4	5
Other Medical		25	25	15–20

[a] These figures assume no treatment to correct the congenital disorders. Approximately one-third of congenital malformations, however, are easily corrected, with no remaining handicap to the child. Assuming optimum treatment, by age 8–9, only 3 percent of children would still have congenital chronic conditions requiring care.

Table 10.

Estimated Numbers and Proportions of Children
With Handicapping Conditions, 1965

Conditions	Estimated Number Handicapped	Age Group	Estimated Proportion Handicapped
Eye Conditions Needing Specialist Care	11,404,000	5–17	23%
Emotionally Disturbed	4,600,000	5–19	8.5
Speech Disorders	2,829,000	5–20	5
Mentally Retarded[a]	2,440,000	0–20	3
Orthopedic	2,153,000	0–20	2.8
Hearing Impairments	2,130,000	0–20	2.8
Cerebral Palsy[b]	406,000	0–20	0.5
Epilepsy	400,000	0–20	0.5

[a] Only one-tenth of these are more than mildly retarded (estimate by National Association of Retarded Children).
[b] It is estimated by the Children's Bureau that 60 to 70 percent of the children with cerebral palsy are mentally retarded.
Source: Children's Bureau, 1966 (percentages added).

Table 11.

Chronic Handicapping Conditions in 18-Year-Olds, and Proportions Preventable or Correctable by Therapy

Diagnosis	Proportion of 18-Year-Olds Chronically Handicapped[a]	Proportion Preventable or Correctable Through Comprehensive Health Care[b]		Proportion Preventable or Correctable Through Case-Finding and Treatment at Ages 0, 1, 3, 5, and 9
		Up to Age 5	Up to Age 15	
Orthopedic-Musculoskeletal	2.38%	15%	45%	25%
Asthma	0.81	40	75	20
Hernia	0.66	27	81	45
Genitourinary	0.35	5	82	78
Rheumatic Heart Disease	0.22	0	78	5
Congenital Heart Disease	0.15	20	35	30
Epilepsy	0.13	55	79	66
Diabetes	0.11	8	64	5
Avitaminosis	0.10	30	54	15
Dental	0.09	28	72	N.A.
Tuberculosis	0.04	45	81	76
Subtotal for Diagnoses Shown	5.04	20	60	30
Total for All Diagnoses (except vision, hearing, and failure to meet anthropometric standards)[c]	12.23			
Eye Problems	0.78	76	85	75
Ear and Mastoid	0.72	47	85	20
Hearing Acuity	0.69	27	50	25
Visual Acuity	0.56	27	29	20
Total for Diagnoses Shown	7.78	30	62	33
Total for All Diagnoses (except failure to meet anthropometric standards)[c]	15.27			

[a] Preliminary data based on rejection rates in special Selective Service examinations of 18-year-old, noncollege-bound youth (July 1964–December 1965) under the Conservation of Manpower program (Source: Dr. Bernard Karpinos, Office of the Surgeon General, Department of the Army).
[b] Rough estimates of the effects of good health care, based on a survey of the medical literature on these leading handicapping conditions. Conditions corrected are conditions not handicapping in civilian life.
[c] Failure to meet anthropometric standards (underheight, underweight—excluding malnutrition, overheight, overweight) accounted for rejection of an additional 3.17 percent of these 18-year-olds.

Table 12.

Percent of Children Ages 5 to 14 With No Visits to Dentists
During the Year June 1963-June 1964

Total (All Races)	45.1%
White	40.4
Nonwhite	73.9
Total (All Family Incomes)	45.1
Under $2,000/year	78.7
$2,000–$3,999	65.2
$4,000–$6,999	47.8
$7,000–$9,999	34.0
Over $10,000	20.1
Total (All Regions)	45.1
Northeast	33.9
North Central	39.0
South	59.7
West	44.4

children not receiving needed dental care: nearly 60 percent of children in the South, more than 65 percent of children in low-income families, and more than 70 percent of nonwhite children are receiving inadequate (or no) dental care.

Cost and Effectiveness of Maternal and Child Health Care Programs

Interrelationships among the effects of environment, education, and medical care make it quite difficult to predict what kind of health improvements will result from improvements in health care delivery; the results of health care programs usually are not measurable for some years. This analysis estimates, however, that health care can significantly improve the health of children in health-depressed areas by reducing both mortality and chronic handicapping conditions. The total cost, manpower requirements, and estimated effects of 12 possible child health care programs were addressed in the analysis under the following major headings:

1. Comprehensive Maternal and Child Health Care Programs.
2. Programs to Provide Early Case-Finding and Treatment of Congenital and Other Chronic Disorders.

3. Programs to Provide Early Case-Finding and Treatment of Vision and Hearing Defects.
4. Programs to Reduce Unmet Dental Needs.
5. Intensive Care Units for High-Risk Premature and Other Newborn Infants.
6. Programs of Support for Expanded Family Planning Services.

To allow for meaningful comparison of program costs and effects, whenever possible, the projected impact of the programs is examined in a health-depressed urban or rural community of 50,000 persons, including 1,000 expectant mothers, 1,000 infants, 1,000 1-year-olds, and 1,000 18-year-olds. The following are brief descriptions of each of the alternatives.

1. Comprehensive Maternal and Child Health Care Programs.

   1.1 Comprehensive care for 1,000 mothers and 18,000 children under 18 years of age, with maximum use of new categories of health personnel (obstetric assistants, pediatric assistants, and dental auxiliaries).
   1.2 Comprehensive care for 1,000 mothers and 18,000 children under 18 years of age, using only traditional health personnel.
   1.3 Comprehensive health care for 1,000 mothers and 5,000 children under five years of age, with maximum use of new categories of health personnel (as in 1.1 above).
   1.4 Comprehensive care for 1,000 mothers and 5,000 children under five years of age, using only traditional health personnel.

2. Programs to Provide Early Case-Finding and Treatment of Congenital and Other Chronic Disorders.

   2.1 Screening, follow-up, and treatment of newborn infants in health-depressed areas. Since many newborns currently do not receive a thorough pediatric evaluation, diagnosis and treatment of congenital and other disorders are delayed, occasionally until a life-threatening situation exists. Newborns can be examined prior to hospital discharge, preferably at age three to five days.
   2.2 Case-finding and treatment for children in health-depressed areas at specified ages; for example, four days, one year, three years, five or six years, and nine years.

3. Programs to Provide Early Case-Finding and Treatment of Vision and Hearing Defects.

   3.1 This is a subprogram of Program 2.2: Early Case-Finding and Treatment of Vision and Hearing Defects. This includes state and local programs in vision and hearing, with screening developed or expanded to include referral and correction of defects so that as many vision and hearing defects as possible may be detected and treated at ages three, five or six, and nine.

4. Programs to Reduce Unmet Dental Needs.

   4.1 Federal grants for the installation of fluoride equipment for community water supply, plus annual financial bonuses to help meet the costs of operating and maintaining fluoridation programs.
   4.2 Comprehensive dental care to school children in grades 1 to 12. Dental services would include diagnosis; prophylaxis; fillings; extractions; typical fluoride applications, where necessary; and tooth-space maintainers.
   4.3 This is a combination of 4.1 and 4.2.

5. Intensive Care Units for High-Risk Premature and Other Infants.

   5.1 Encompasses facilitating the development of intensive care centers for high-risk premature and other newborns.

6. Expanded Family Planning Services.

   6.1 Makes available voluntary family planning programs to those who would not otherwise have access to such services. Included are project grants awarded to public and private nonprofit agencies for developing or improving family planning programs that are an integral part of maternal or other health services for women in health-depressed areas. Such programs would include dissemination of family planning information, services, and supplies to any woman seeking such services.

Cost and Effectiveness of Achieving the Proposed Objectives

The cost and effectiveness data are summarized in Table 13. The analytical task is to select those programs and quantities thereof that are preferred, based on their relative efficiency.[4]

It is immediately clear from Table 13 that, of the comprehensive alternatives, 1.2 is dominated by 1.1,[5] and 1.4 is dominated by 1.3.[6] In each case, where effectiveness is equal, costs are lower for the preferred alternatives. As the two dominated alternatives have no further role, they may be deleted from consideration.[7]

The remaining alternatives in the analysis are now divided into two groups: programs aimed at reducing chronic handicapping conditions (child health care) and programs aimed at reducing conditions associated with maternal health care. In order to accomplish this analysis, the two remaining comprehensive health care alternatives (1.1 and 1.3)—each of which covers both of the groups—are partitioned to conform to each of the two groups. Thus the costs and effectiveness attributable to each group are separately identified. Table 14 separates the costs for mothers from the costs for children.

The alternative programs for child health care are as follows: 1.1—Comprehensive Health Care (children up to age 18), 1.3—Comprehensive Health Care (children up to age 5), and 2.2—Case-Finding and Treatment (ages 0, 1, 3, 5, and 9). Table 14 (which draws data from Table 13) depicts the comparative effectiveness and resource requirements for each of the alternatives. Cost-effectiveness ratios cannot be used, because there is no satisfactory way to either allocate the costs to each of the effectiveness indicators or collapse the effectiveness indicators into a composite measure of utility that can be related to the costs. Lacking this ability, nevertheless, some judgments can be made about the relative preference for the alternatives. Clearly, Case-Finding and Treatment (ages 0, 1, 3, 5, and 9) dominates Comprehensive Health Care (children to age 5), because in all the effectiveness categories, the effectiveness is equal to or greater for that alternative, and the costs are substantially lower. Thus, unless the marginal

---

[4] Obviously, when one uses the efficiency criterion, he assumes, at least at that time, that all other factors are equal (or can be ignored).

[5] Both 1.1 and 1.2 are comprehensive health care (mothers and children to age 18).

[6] Both 1.4 and 1.3 are comprehensive health care (mothers and children up to age five).

[7] Unless various constraints require the further consideration of these comparatively inefficient alternatives (for example, the availability of obstetrical assistants).

Table 13.

Summary of Estimated Annual Costs and Effectiveness of Alternative Maternal and Child Health Care Programs in a Health-Depressed Community of 50,000 People

Program	Resource Requirements				Effectiveness				Prevalence of Chronic Handicapping Conditions					
									Uncorrected Vision					
	$000	MD	Dentist	Births	Maternal Deaths	Premature Births	Infant Deaths	Mentally Retarded	All	Amblyopia	All	Binaural	Other Physical Handicaps	Unmet Dental Needs
1.1 Comprehensive Health Care (mothers and children up to age 18)	2,896	11.7	4	—	.45	28–69	12–17	1–2	100	17	35	2.1	58	650
1.2 Comprehensive Health Care (mothers and children up to age 18)	3,054	22.5	11	—	.45	28–29	12–17	1–2	100	17	35	2.1	58	650
1.3 Comprehensive Health Care (mothers and children up to age 5)	1,429	6.8	1	—	.45	28–29	12–17	1–2	28	17	10	.7	9	—
1.4 Comprehensive Health Care (mothers and children up to age 5)	1,468	12.6	2	—	.45	28–29	12–17	1–2	28	17	10	.7	9	—
2.1 Case-Finding and Treatment (newborns only)	29.7	.2	—	—	—	—	a	a	—	—	—	—	a	—
2.2 Case-Finding and Treatment (ages 0, 1, 3, 5, and 9)	149.7	13	—	—	—	—	a	a	54	17	15	.9	22	—
3.1 Vision and Hearing Case-Finding and Treatment	20.6	.2	—	—	—	—	—	—	54	17	15	.9	—	—
4.1 Fluoridation	8.5	—	—	—	—	—	—	—	—	—	—	—	—	150
4.2 Comprehensive Dental Care (without Fluoridation)	270	—	2.5	—	—	—	—	—	—	—	—	—	—	400
4.3 Comprehensive Dental Care (plus Fluoridation)	125.5	—	1.3	—	—	—	—	—	—	—	—	—	—	463
5.1 Intensive Care Units for High-Risk Newborns	49.1	.2	—	—	—	—	5	a	—	—	—	—	—	—
6.1 Expanded Family Planning Services	3.2	—	—	170	.1	a	16	8.5	—	—	—	—	—	—

a Some improvements are anticipated, no quantitative estimates were made.

Table 14.

Reduction in Prevalence of Chronic Handicapping Conditions—
Programs Serving Health-Depressed Community of 50,000 People

	Comprehen-sive Health Care to Age 18 (1.1)	Comprehen-sive Health Care to Age 5 (1.3)	Case-Finding and Treatment (0, 1, 3, 5 and 9) (2.2)
Vision Problems[a]			
All	100	28	54
Amblyopia	17	17	17
All[a]	25	10	15
Binaural[a]	2.1	.7	.9
Other Physical Handicaps[a]	58	9	22
Unmet Dental Needs[a]	650	0	0
Program Cost ($000)	2,900	1,430	150
Cost for Mothers	560	560	—
Cost for Children	2,340	870	150
MD's Required[a]	11.7	6.8	1.3
Dentists Required[a]	4.0	1.0	0

[a] Number.

cost-effectiveness curves for larger programs are substantially dissimilar, this program should be pursued to the maximum extent feasible.[8] The selection between Comprehensive Health Care (children up to age 5) and Comprehensive Health Care (children up to age 18) depends upon the relative values the decision maker attaches to the various effectiveness categories.

In the case of programs aimed at other than chronic handicapping conditions, the major alternatives are: Comprehensive Health Care to age 18, Comprehensive Health Care to age 5, Intensive Care Units for High-Risk Newborns, and Expanded Family Planning Services. Table 15 depicts the comparative effectiveness and costs of the alternatives. Clearly, Expanded Family Planning Services is dominant, as it equals or exceeds the effectiveness of the alternatives while costing substantially less (except that it falls into the upper range of two of the alternatives for reducing infant deaths). Both of the Comprehensive Health Care alternatives are exactly equal, as their

[8] There are, of course, substantial differences in magnitude among the alternatives ($2,000, $340,000, $870,000, and $150,000). Thus, the comparison could be misleading for the same reasons as apply to benefit-cost ratios. Therefore, a second step should be to examine the three alternatives at alternative fixed budget levels of (say) $10, $50, and $100 million.

Table 15.

Reduction in Prevalence of Conditions Associated with Inadequate
Maternal Care—Programs Serving Health-Depressed Community
of 50,000 People

	Compre-hensive Health Care (to age 18) (1.1)	Compre-hensive Health Care (to age 5) (1.3)	Intensive Care Units for High-Risk Newborns (5.1)	Expanded Family Planning Services (6.1)
Births[a]	0	0	0	170
Maternal Deaths[a]	0.45	0.45	0	0.8
Premature Births[a]	28–69	28–69	0	Some Im-provement
Infant Deaths[a]	12–17	12–17	5	16
Mentally Retarded[a]	1–2	1–2	Some Im-provement	8.5
Program Costs ($000)	2,900	1,430	49	32
Cost for Children	2,340	870	—	—
Cost for Mothers	560	560	49	32
MD's Required[a]	11.7	6.8	0.2	—
Dentists Required[a]	4.0	1.0	0	—

[a] Number.

costs and effectiveness (for mothers) are identical. The selection between
the Comprehensive Health Care alternatives and the Intensive Care Units
depends upon the decision maker's relative preference.

Table 16 depicts the comparative effectiveness, resource requirements,
and effectiveness/cost ratios of alternative programs to reduce unmet dental
needs. In this case, resource inputs and effectiveness outputs each are single
measures; thus, jointness of cost and product is not a factor. In this case,
effectiveness/cost ratios may be used to determine the comparative efficiency
of the alternatives. It is immediately clear from the comparative preference
ratios that Fluoridation (4.1) is dominant, Comprehensive Dental Care plus
Fluoridation (4.3) is next, and Comprehensive Dental Care without Fluoridation (4.2) is last. There are wide differences in the absolute magnitude of
the comparative costs; both should be examined at alternative fund levels.
Significantly higher reductions in unmet dental needs can be attained by

Table 16.

Reduction in Unmet Dental Needs—Programs Servicing
Health-Depressed Community of 50,000 People

	Fluoridation (4.1)	Comprehensive Dental Care without Fluoridation (4.2)	Comprehensive Dental Care with Fluoridation (4.3)
Reduction	150	400	463
E/C Ratio	.057	.67	.27
Program Costs ($000)	8.5	270	125.5
Dentists Required[a]	0	2.5	1.3

[a] Number.

pursuing less efficient programs. The decision maker could believe, for example, that it is worth the additional cost to pursue 4.3 and achieve a much
larger reduction (463 compared to 150) in unmet dental needs.

Thus far, we have grouped programs sharing common effectiveness measures and have determined the dominant ones within each group. The alternative programs may be ranked on an ordinal scale as shown in Table 17.
This scale depicts the relative rankings, based on the cost-effectiveness
criteria of programs with similar effectiveness objectives. Such criteria, however, are not very useful for choosing among programs having substantially
different objectives. Thus, the choice among programs to reduce chronic
handicapping conditions, unmet dental needs, and other needs depends upon
the decision maker's relative preference. This type of procedure will provide

Table 17.

Ordinal Rankings of Alternative Programs
by Program Category

Ordinal Preference	Chronic Handicapping Conditions	Unmet Dental Needs	Other
1	2.2	4.1	6.1
2	1.1	4.3	1.1, 1.3, 5.1
3	1.3	4.2	

Table 18.

Benefit/Cost Ratios for Alternative Maternal and Child Health Care—
Programs for a Community of 50,000 People

Alternative	Benefits (thousands $)	Costs (thousands $)	Benefits/ Costs
1.1 Comprehensive Health Care (up to age 18— new personnel)	10,410	2,896	3.6
1.2 Comprehensive Health Care (up to age 18— traditional personnel)	10,410	3,054	3.4
1.3 Comprehensive Health Care (up to age 5— new personnel)	4,717	1,429	3.3
1.4 Comprehensive Health Care (up to age 5— traditional personnel)	4,717	1,469	3.2
2.1 Case-Finding and Treatment (newborns)	1,174	29.7	39.5
2.2 Case-Finding and Treatment (age 0, 1, 3, 5, 9)	4,561	149.7	30.5

Source: David Kendrick, *A Benefit-Cost Analysis of Maternal and Child Health Care Programs*, Washington, D.C., Program Evaluation Staff, Bureau of the Budget, 1967.

a far superior basis for decision making than will merely presenting the unassembled costs and effectiveness of the alternatives.[9]

Cost-benefit comparisons also might have a role in providing the decision maker with information concerning the economic payoffs of the alternatives. Confronted with such an apparently significant disparity in benefit-cost ratios among the comprehensive and other alternatives shown in Table 18, the decision maker might consider this additional information quite useful in making his decision. Such measures have the advantage of collapsing effectiveness streams and allowing comparisons among programs having dissimilar objectives and effectiveness measures. The decision maker should be aware of the shortcomings intrinsic to benefit-cost analysis and should carefully

[9] This might be influenced to varying degrees by the decision maker's background (for example, a pediatrician might be most concerned with chronic handicapping conditions), the agency's priorities (for example, if reducing infant mortality is a top priority, comprehensive maternal care becomes more attractive), and political and institutional factors (for example, family planning may be politically most acceptable while the medical profession opposes the use of pediatric assistants).

examine the reasoning and assumptions that caused such large differences in the ratios.[10]

The comparative costs, effectiveness, and benefits do not, however, exhaust the information of interest to the decision maker. He is also interested in the costs of other scarce resources—notably MD's and dentists. Thus, additional rows in Tables 15 and 16 were included to depict the requirements of each alternative. These act as constraints in determining the preferred solution.

The decision maker also is concerned about the extent to which the program expenditures proposed for these alternatives would replace expenditures now incurred by the nonfederal sectors.

Another critical element in his criteria is the question of political support for the programs. Thus, the impact by state, congressional district, and client group is quite relevant to his decision.

Conclusions

This case has illustrated a "classical" application of policy analysis. It proceeded in a series of steps essentially conforming to those suggested in Part I of this book.

Based on the alternatives presented in this analysis, the decision maker should be particularly interested in the following programs:

1. Case-finding and treatment.
2. Family planning.
3. Possibly one of the dental care alternatives.

In addition, if he desires to meet the comprehensive health care objectives, he also might consider one of those alternatives.

---

[10] If both effectiveness/cost and benefit/cost analysis are used, the decision maker should realize the overlap between them—benefits and effectiveness are not mutually additive. Note also the limitations in ratios previously discussed.

CHAPTER 5

SIMULATION AND COST-EFFECTIVENESS ANALYSIS OF NEW YORK'S EMERGENCY AMBULANCE SERVICE[1]

Introduction

Since 1870, the City of New York has been providing emergency ambulance service to its residents and visitors. With the growth of the city, the service is now available to approximately 10 million persons daily, 24 hours a day, every day of the year. In 1967, the city's ambulance service responded to more than half a million calls for emergency assistance, an increase of more than 43 percent in the past decade. This growing workload, together with an increasing concern about the adequacy and responsiveness of the system, led to a request by the mayor to analyze the service and to recommend and implement significant improvements.

Scope of the Study

EMERGENCY MEDICAL CARE—AN OVERVIEW

Viewed in perspective, the emergency ambulance service fits within the more general framework of an overall emergency medical care system. Such a system is composed of the following subsystems, with the first two comprising what is usually considered the ambulance system: communication, transportation, and medical treatment.

Preventive health care also enters into the total picture, for it clearly affects the requirements for, and the nature of, an emergency medical care system. Improved preventive health measures and their ready availability to the community (for example, through Neighborhood Health Care Centers) can be expected to reduce the demand for emergency care.

---

[1] This case is based on the work of E. S. Savas, Deputy City Administrator, City of New York. It was originally written by Richard J. Gill and modified slightly for this book.

Communication Subsystem: Includes the means by which help is summoned for a patient, and the procedures for screening, assessing, and establishing priorities for such calls. It also encompasses the requirements and means for communication among dispatchers, ambulances, and hospitals, and possibly even for contacting the Doctor's Emergency Service, Poison Control Center, etc.

Transportation Subsystem: Includes the means for conveying a patient to the medical facility, or for transporting medical facilities (doctor, first-aid attendant, oxygen, resuscitation equipment, stomach pump, antidotes, etc.) to a patient. Elements within this subsystem include such factors as the boundaries of ambulance service districts, the locations of ambulances and hospitals, and the number of ambulances. Other elements might involve the use of sirens and express lanes, the design and construction of ambulances, the location of first-aid stations, and devices for carrying people down stairs.

Medical Treatment Subsystem: This area encompasses the nature, speed, and adequacy of emergency medical treatment: that is, the qualifications of personnel; their prompt availability; the organization, procedures, and equipment in an emergency room; the equipment carried in an ambulance; the possible utility of first-aid stations, etc. The life-saving value of improvements in the transportation subsystem could be vitiated, for example, if no doctor were available immediately after the patient is carried into the hospital.

ANALYSIS OF THE EMERGENCY AMBULANCE SERVICE

Due to the urgent need to improve the ambulance service itself, no effort was made initially to examine the prevention or treatment subsystems; the major effort was focused on particular elements of the transportation subsystem. Specifically, a quantitative analysis was made of the geographic distribution of emergency calls in the most severe problem area of the city and of the number and placement of ambulances needed to service these calls effectively. The merits of a proposed satellite ambulance station were examined in detail.

Objective: The concept of improved ambulance service can be described quantitatively by two related performance measures:

Response time—the period between receipt of a call at the ambulance station and arrival of an ambulance at the scene.

Round-trip time—the period between receipt of a call at the ambulance station and arrival of the assigned ambulance at the hospital with the patient.

Both of these related parameters are important from the public service point of view. Prompt arrival of an ambulance and a trained attendant on the scene saves lives, reduces suffering, and produces confidence in the service by the general citizenry. Round-trip time is the vital parameter whereby the patient requires prompt, professional medical treatment in the emergency room of a hospital.

The objective adopted in the Kings County Hospital district of Brooklyn was to decrease the response time. (It follows from the above definitions that a decrease in response time produces the same reduction in round-trip time.) However, no numerical target (for example, a five-minute reduction in response time) could justifiably be set unless it were possible to relate time savings to the saving of lives. No such study has been reported, and to tackle this problem was well outside the initial scope of the project; it remains an important topic for future medical research.

Alternatives: The following three alternatives were considered initially:

1. Redistribute the existing ambulances in the district by locating some of them at a satellite garage.
2. Increase the number of ambulances at Kings County Hospital.
3. A combination of the previous two alternatives.

Criteria: Both the cost and the effectiveness of the alternatives were considered. Costs included the capital outlay and the operating costs of additional ambulances and of a satellite garage. Effectiveness was measured by minutes of average response time and also by the percentage of calls whose response time exceeded a certain level.

THE PROBLEM

Figure 10 portrays a typical district served by a hospital, indicated by H in the figure. Under the present mode of operation, all of the ambulances serving that district are stationed at the hospital. The dots on the map indi-

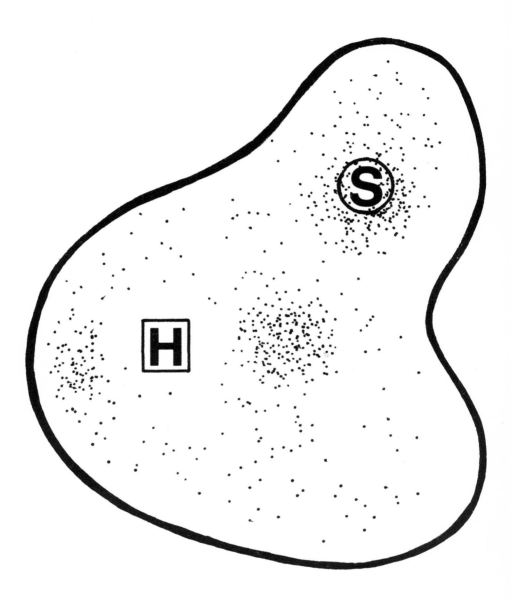

Figure 10. General representation of an ambulance district, showing locations of hospital, H, satellite garage, S, and points where calls were made.

cate the locations and relative numbers of emergency calls from different points throughout the district. Calls are not uniformly and randomly distributed throughout the area. Due to varying population distribution and socioeconomic characteristics, certain subsections of the district exhibit a rather dense clustering of dots; that is, there is a high demand for ambulance service in those areas.

A superficial look at Figure 10 suggests that a substantial improvement in ambulance service could be achieved by the relatively simple expedient of stationing ambulances at a satellite garage in the middle of one of the clusters, for example, at point S. Such a garage could consist of space in an ordinary commercial garage, or could be the garage of a police station or firehouse. Proponents of this idea reasoned that an ambulance located at the satellite station could pick up a patient in that vicinity and deliver him to the hospital in half the time that it would take an ambulance to go from the hospital, pick up the patient, and return with him to the hospital. They envisioned a 50-percent reduction in round-trip time. A closer look, however, shows that the situation is not so simple. First, not all the elapsed time can be attributed to travel. Various delays contribute to the total round-trip time (see Figure 11), and these delays would not be reduced by relocating the ambulances. Second, the ambulances would be called upon to service calls from anywhere in the district, not only those calls from the immediate vicinity of their satellite station, and it is difficult to forecast an improvement in handling those calls. Finally, the round-trip time is very sensitive to the frequency of calls. For example, infrequent calls from the area around the satellite station could be assigned to waiting ambulances, resulting in a substantial improvement. If, however, the frequency of calls were to increase, the ambulances would be spending more and more time shuttling back and forth between the hospital and the high-demand area around the satellite station, and calls would queue up to await an available ambulance, in which case it would make no difference where the busy ambulance was stationed—at the satellite garage, at the hospital, or at any point in between.

This qualitative analysis clearly shows that the picture is not so simple as it appears at first glance, and that the level of service depends, in a complex way, on the following five major factors: geographic distribution of calls throughout the district, frequency of calls, number of ambulances in the district, location of the hospital, and location of ambulance garage(s).

Given the complexity of this system, no intuitive estimate can provide a sound guide. Nevertheless, the basic idea of a satellite station—to put the

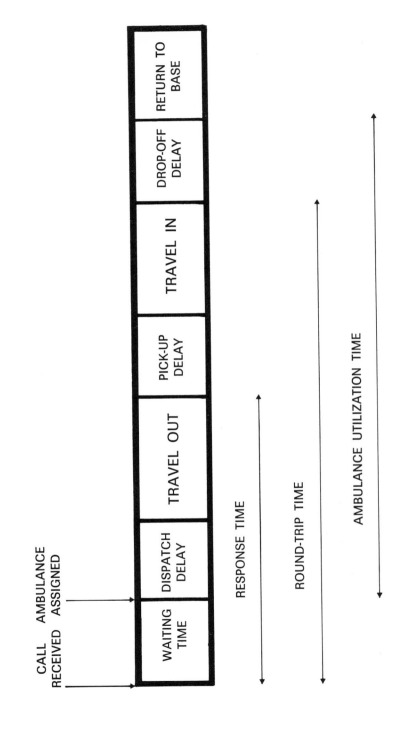

Figure 11. Sequence of events during a call, showing time relationships.

ambulances where they are needed—is a sound one that warrants a detailed, quantitative analysis in order to provide valid estimates of the improvements that can be expected.

THE APPROACH

Since the level of service is a complicated function of five variables, conventional computational approaches and simple mathematics will not suffice. Instead, the ideal analytical tool would be computer simulation. Computer simulation is particularly effective when problems involve many interrelated factors, when the expected effects are complex, and when trial-and-error experimentation is costly or impractical.

Ambulance service in the Kings County Hospital district was simulated on a digital computer using a mathematical model of the system. A map of the district, as of August 1966, appears in Figure 12. The hospital is located at H; the proposed satellite, at S. About 175,000 calls were simulated, corresponding to almost four years of operation of that hospital's ambulance service. Attention was focused on the peak-load period—the 4 p.m.-to-midnight shift. The inter-arrival time was set at 7.28 minutes, which characterized the peak-load period in an average month of 4,570 calls. (This number of calls was 15 percent greater than the actual observed monthly load, to allow for the predicted future load.) General and technical details concerning the simulation appear elsewhere.[2] A general flow diagram of the model appears in Figure 13.

Results of the Simulation

EFFECT OF A SATELLITE STATION

Seven ambulances were retained to service the Kings County Hospital district, and the effect of a satellite station at the location indicated in Figure 12 was simulated. Figure 14 illustrates how the average round-trip time and average response time are affected as the seven ambulances are redistributed between the hospital and the satellite station in various proportions.

[2] G. Gordon and K. Zelin. "A Simulation Study of Emergency Ambulance Service in New York City." New York, IBM Corporation, 1968. Technical Report No. 320–2935.

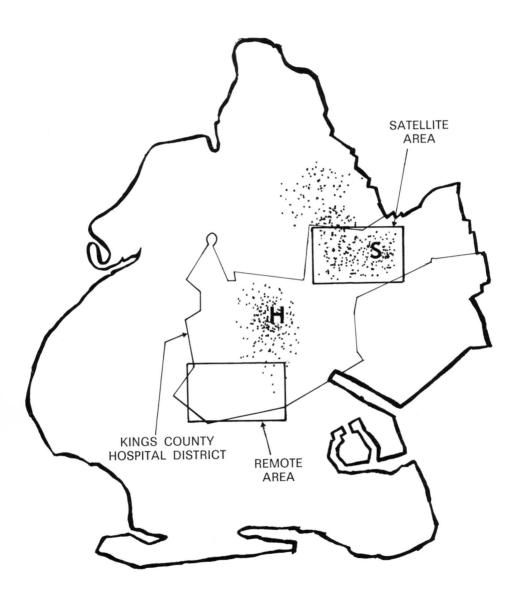

Figure 12. Map of Brooklyn, New York showing hospital district and areas near hospital and satellite.

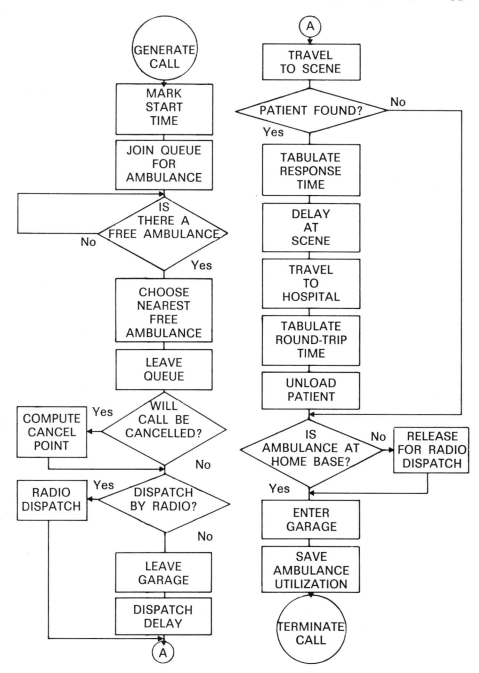

Figure 13. General flow diagram of model.

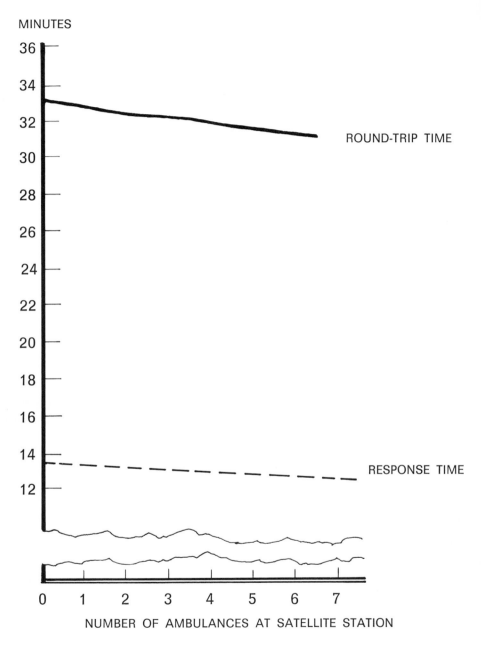

Figure 14. Effect of satellite on service, with a total of seven ambulances in the system.

First, note that both the average round-trip time and the average response time decrease continuously as each ambulance is removed from the hospital and is placed at the satellite garage. Actually, the optimum way to use the available ambulances would be to have all of them located at the satellite and none at the hospital. In other words, the satellite is at a better location than is the hospital itself, at least in terms of ambulance service. This finding should not be interpreted as an argument for moving the hospital. A constructive conclusion is that redrawing the hospital district lines, as well as redeployment of ambulances, may be in order.

The second conclusion to be drawn from Figure 14 is a disappointing one: the average round-trip time is reduced a mere 5 percent—from 33 to 31.5 minutes—which is far less than the 50-percent improvement that seemed so obvious at first glance. (This reduction of 1.5 minutes applies to the average response time as well, and constitutes an 11-percent improvement over the existing time of 13.5 minutes.)

EFFECT OF ADDITIONAL AMBULANCES

Here, the effect of placing additional ambulances at the hospital was studied. The results are evident in Figure 15. Average response time drops by 0.3 minutes as the number of ambulances stationed at the hospital is increased from 7 to 10; but, thereafter, virtually no improvement occurs, no matter how many ambulances are added. Only one reaches the elbow of the curve, one is operating on a plateau, and additional ambulances are wasted. This is an excellent example of "diminishing returns."

Waiting Time: In Figure 16, the solid line shows the average waiting time as it relates to the number of ambulances at the hospital. Waiting time is the period between receipt of a call at the ambulance station and assignment of an available ambulance to service that call (see Figure 11). Waiting time constitutes one identifiable segment of the response time. As more ambulances are added to the system, the waiting time drops essentially to zero, and the response time levels off (see Figure 15), depending almost exclusively on the travel time. Travel time is a fixed characteristic of a given district and depends upon its geometry (size and shape, and the location of its ambulances) and its traffic (routes and conditions).

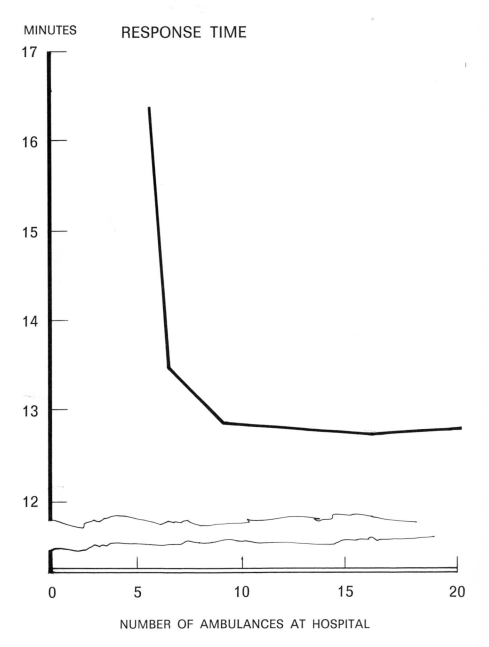

MINUTES   RESPONSE TIME

17

16

15

14

13

12

0   5   10   15   20

NUMBER OF AMBULANCES AT HOSPITAL

Figure 15. Effect on response time of additional ambulances at the hospital.

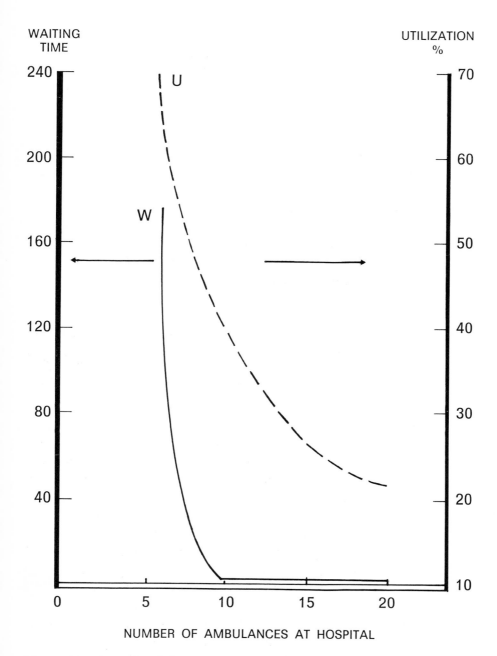

Figure 16. Effect of additional ambulances on waiting time and on ambulance utilization.

Ambulance Utilization: The broken line in Figure 16 shows how ambulance utilization declines as more ambulances are added. (Utilization is the fraction of time that an ambulance spends on a call; see Figure 11 for a graphic definition.) The increase in idle time (decreased utilization) is the penalty for reducing the average waiting time, that is, for assurance that an ambulance will be available for prompt assignment when a call comes in.

It should be noted that the minimum response (at the elbow of Figure 15) —which is achieved when the waiting time approaches zero (see Figure 16)— corresponds to a utilization of 42 percent. This compares to the actual current utilization of about 60 percent.

This utilization factor is an important indicator of service and, because it is relatively easy to measure, can be used to manage the ambulance system. For example, given the existing boundaries for Kings County Hospital (with no satellite station), this analysis shows that, if utilization is greater than 42 percent, improved service can be obtained by adding ambulances. On the other hand, if utilization is less than 42 percent, ambulances can safely be released from the district without fear that the level of service will deteriorate. Furthermore, simple arithmetic suffices to calculate how many ambulances to add or remove in order to arrive at the 42-percent utilization figure.

Economy of Large Districts: Figure 17 displays the relationship between workload (in calls per month) and ideal utilization (the utilization corresponding to negligible waiting time, for example, 42 percent). The significant observation here is that ideal utilization is not constant and independent of the load; as the load increases, the ideal utilization rate also increases. In other words, if the load were to be doubled, one would need less than twice as many ambulances in order to continue providing ideal service. This result has important policy ramifications. It means that a group of small districts, each with a small load and one or two ambulances, requires more ambulances to provide a given level of service than would be required if the districts were consolidated into a single large district with the ambulances pooled under a unified command. The same effect is achieved by ignoring district lines and simply assigning the nearest available ambulance.

Figure 17 could be used to adjust the number of ambulances in the Kings County Hospital district as the workload fluctuates over time. With minor modification, the data also could be used to guide the staffing patterns of the three work shifts.

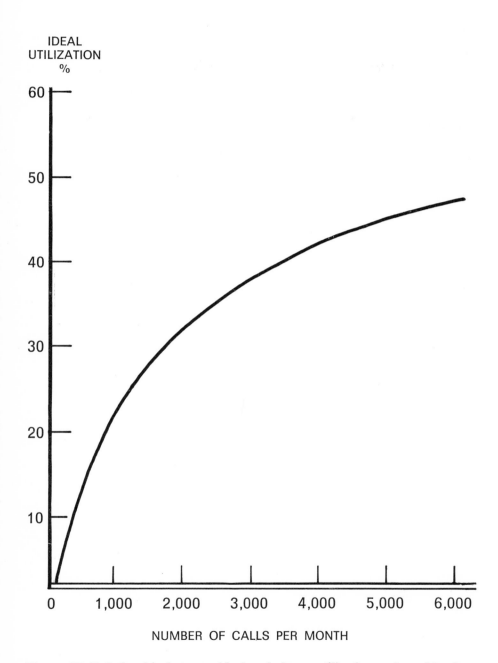

Figure 17. Relationship between ideal ambulance utilization and workload.

EFFECT OF A SATELLITE STATION WITH ADDITIONAL AMBULANCES
The number of ambulances serving the district was increased to 10, and their effect, with a satellite station, was simulated.

Figure 18 shows the results for various distributions of the 10 ambulances between the hospital and the satellite station. The corresponding curve for seven ambulances, taken from Figure 14, is also shown for comparative purposes.

The most important feature to observe is that the response time drops to a minimum of 10.9 minutes (with six ambulances at the satellite station and four at the hospital), a reduction of 19 percent from the pre-existing 13.5 minute average. When more than six ambulances are at the satellite station, the service gets worse; that is, the area near the satellite becomes over-saturated with ambulances. Too many ambulances at the hospital also wastes resources.

Service in Subareas: Thus far, the discussion has centered on average response time for the entire district. The next question is whether certain subareas of the district would experience a *decline* in service; a decline that might be masked in the district average because of a more-than-compensating improvement in service in the subarea near the satellite. Accordingly, the remote subarea and the satellite subarea indicated by the two rectangular areas on the map in Figure 12 were examined. The results are shown in Figure 19. As would be expected, the satellite subarea has better service than the district average; with the six ambulances at the satellite station, the satellite subarea has an average response time of 10.0 minutes, a 21-percent improvement over its pre-existing value of 12.8 minutes. Even for the remote subarea, it was gratifying to note an improvement of 6 percent over the pre-existing situation; a drop from 16.1 to 15.1 minutes when the ambulances are divided 4/6 between the hospital and the satellite station.

Proposed System

On the basis of the simulation results, it was concluded that the proposed satellite station, with additional ambulances, could be justified as an immediate way to realize substantial improvements. This satellite was placed in operation on a pilot basis; however, it was felt that further improvements were possible.

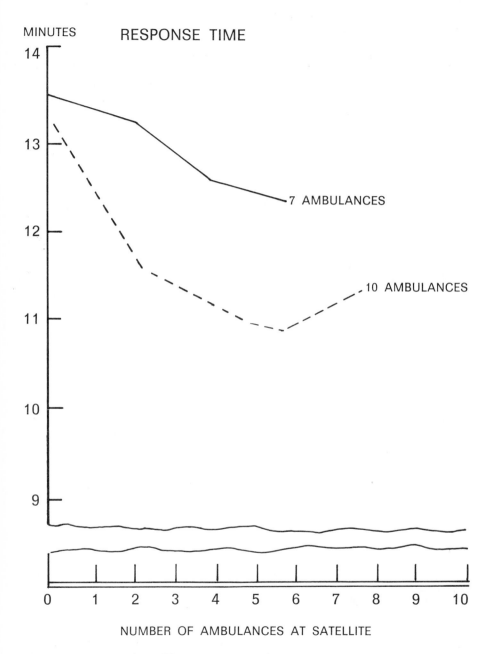

Figure 18. Effect of satellite on response time.

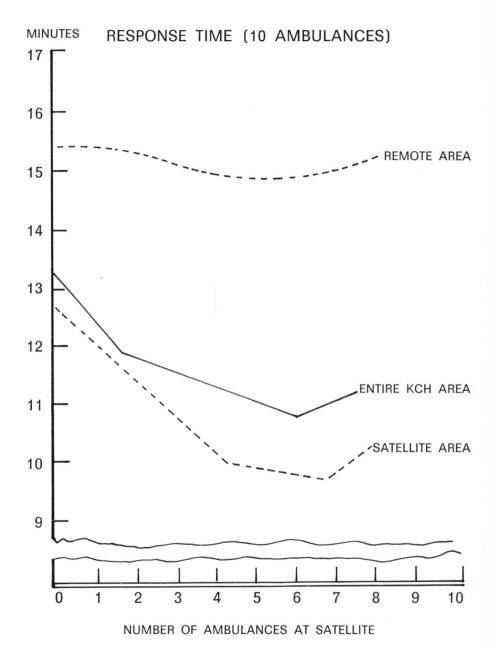

MINUTES   RESPONSE TIME (10 AMBULANCES)

REMOTE AREA

ENTIRE KCH AREA

SATELLITE AREA

NUMBER OF AMBULANCES AT SATELLITE

Figure 19. Effect of satellite on service to remote area and to area near satellite.

It was previously stated that Kings County Hospital is not particularly well-situated within the district that its ambulances service. Undoubtedly, this is true of many other districts in the city as well. This suggests that one improvement would be to redistrict the city, taking into consideration the locations of the hospitals and the distribution of calls in order to draw more rational district boundaries.

In considering this suggestion, however, a different and more fundamental recommendation emerged: *ambulances ought to be stationed where the patients are* without regard to hospital locations, and *an ambulance ought to bring a patient to the nearest appropriate treatment center* without regard to the ambulance's home station. In other words, the transportation and the treatment subsystems should be separated (decoupled). The problems, therefore, can be stated as: where to locate ambulances so they reach patients promptly; and where to deliver patients.

LOCATION OF AMBULANCES

From a practical standpoint, the recommendation to divorce the transportation service from the treatment service means that ambulances should be operated centrally, for example, by the Department of Hospitals. They should be distributed throughout the city in accordance with the observed demand, and they should be redistributed periodically as the geographic pattern of demand is modified due to changes in the population. Hospitals are relatively permanent installations with no mobility; therefore, it makes little sense for the transportation service to be attached so inflexibly to such facilities.

These statements should not be interpreted to mean that ambulances should not be stationed at hospitals. If the distribution of calls indicates that a particular hospital is so situated that it can serve as an ambulance station, it should be used as such.

It is evident that, to reduce response time, ambulances should be completely dispersed; that is, rarely should there be two or more ambulances stationed at one location. The simulation clearly showed how the response time improves as existing ambulances from one station are apportioned properly between two stations to put them closer to high-demand areas. Further dissemination will result in further improvement, and the maximum decentralization—one ambulance per station—should produce the maximum improvement. This statement is in no way inconsistent with the previous statement concerning the economy of large districts. The crucial point here is the elimination of the entire concept of districts so far as the transportation subsystem is concerned. The nearest available ambulance will be assigned to a call, without regard to any real or hypothetical district boundaries. This approach is completely equivalent to making the entire city a single district and having all the ambulances serve that district. This is in perfect harmony with the comments about the savings in time associated with large, multi-ambulance districts.

It has been shown that satellite garages, provided they are committed to only short-term leases and amortization of capital conversion costs, offer one relatively inexpensive way of providing a more rational dispersion and distribution of ambulances; however, a further extension of this concept is suggested. It is not clear whether ambulances must be kept inside a garage while awaiting assignment. Just as there are taxi stands, bus stops, and reserved parking places in front of hotels, consulates, hospitals, and post offices, one can conceive of on-the-street ambulance stations. In addition to permitting optimal placement of ambulances, this would reduce costs, increase the visibility of the service, and probably reduce the dispatching delay. (On the other hand, additional unnecessary calls might be generated by virtue of the high visibility.) The problem of comfort facilities for the ambulance crew can be handled the same as it is handled for radio patrolmen, bus drivers, sanitation men, and taxi drivers. In the winter, the problem of keeping warm in a standing ambulance should be surmountable; at worst, it would be necessary to keep the motor running, although this could prove costly in gasoline and in contributing to noise and air pollution.

Dispatching of ambulances in such a highly decentralized system must be performed centrally, as it is now being performed by the Communications Bureau of the Police Department, but without going through an intermediary dispatcher at a garage. This capability already exists. Each ambulance is equipped with a two-way radio and is in communication with the police dispatcher. The forthcoming computer-based command-and-control system (SPRINT) at the Communications Bureau will enable the ambulance dispatcher to provide even closer, minute-by-minute control over the status and activity of each ambulance in the city system. Furthermore, SPRINT will automate the process of selecting and assigning the nearest available ambulance to each call, despite the wide dispersion of ambulances among many individual locations.

In addition, by employing statistical estimates for the length of time that an ambulance is assigned to a call, the computer might even be able to advise the dispatcher whether to assign a call immediately to a relatively distant but available ambulance, or to wait a few minutes for another ambulance— currently on assignment—that is likely to become available at a location sufficiently close to the point of demand to warrant a brief delay in making the assignment.

Supervisory control, as distinguished from dispatching, would be exercised by the Department of Hospitals by matching information reports on each call from the police dispatcher, the ambulance crew, and the hospital emergency room. SPRINT makes such detailed reporting practical, and such reporting is strengthened by the accurate and prompt feedback on ambulance service that the public provides when it calls in to complain that no ambulance has yet arrived on the scene. This opportunity for feedback control, which is absent in cases of routine preventive police patrol and in sanitation trucks, minimizes the need for on-site supervision. If such supervision is deemed necessary, however, it could be performed by a borough commander driving around on inspection, much the same as a district sanitation superintendent.

This tentative recommendation for a garage-free satellite operation requires more careful evaluation in order to determine its feasibility and to see if any necessary functions of a garage have been overlooked. For example, some garage space would still be needed for parking excess ambulances during low-load shifts. In any event, an ambulance from a street station will have to be driven back to a garage at shift changes. Refueling and minor maintenance could be performed there. Locker facilities at that garage would enable the attendants to change into uniforms and to store personal belongings, as they do now.

DELIVERY OF PATIENTS

The above recommendations, when implemented, will tend to minimize the time required for an ambulance to reach the scene (response time). The next question is where to deliver the patient in order to minimize round-trip time. The ideal answer is to deliver him to the nearest appropriate treatment center. (The general term "treatment center" is used here to leave open the possibility of providing some types of emergency medical care at neighborhood health clinics or first-aid centers. The term "hospital" will be used for the sake of convenience, although the above option should be borne in mind.) The appropriateness of a hospital as a delivery point for ambulance patients depends on the following major factors: adequacy of its emergency room; if not a municipal hospital, its selectivity in terms of interesting cases, a patient's economic resources, and other possible factors; and capacity or bed availability.

One area of possible improvement lies in the first factor. If study shows that average round-trip time in an area could be reduced by bringing patients to a hospital which is not qualified at the present time solely because of inadequate emergency room facilities, the possibility, cost, and effectiveness of upgrading those facilities should be explored. (If such a hospital is too small to accept many emergency patients, it should not be considered, as the *average* round-trip time will not show a marked improvement.)

The second factor, a nonmunicipal hospital's policy of selectivity, is outside the realm of practical analysis. Existing hospital district lines in some cases result from such selection criteria. Analysis can serve to identify those hospitals whose participation—or fuller participation—in the system would substantially improve the emergency ambulance service, thereby providing some direction for policy-making officials to negotiate and otherwise bargain with the private institution to secure its participation on mutually acceptable grounds.

It is the third factor, hospital capacity or bed availability, that presents the greatest problem. For the most part, the whole concept of a hospital's ambulance district is a crude attempt to match the hospital's capacity with the expected number of emergency cases in an area. Because it is such a round approximation, patients are sometimes transferred elsewhere when there is no space, and, conversely, overcrowding occurs despite available beds at a nearby hospital. The ideal situation would be for the central dispatcher to have up-to-the-minute information on the actual number of beds available in each hospital in the system, in which case, the following ideal sequence of events would occur:

1. The dispatcher assigns the nearest available ambulance to a call.
2. After picking up the patient, the ambulance driver informs the dispatcher whether hospitalization is required and whether a specialist or particular equipment is needed immediately upon arrival at the hospital (to the extent that he is able to make such determination).

3. If a hospital bed is required, the dispatcher determines the nearest hospital with an available bed.
4. The dispatcher instructs the ambulance to proceed to that hospital.
5. If the driver has requested special aid to be on hand, the dispatcher so advises the hospital.

The Department of Hospitals has already started developing a computer-based bed inventory system covering the municipal hospitals. Depending on the implementation timetable of various recommendations, the inventory could be made available initially to its ambulances and then, as decentralization of ambulances is carried out, the dispatcher at the Communications Bureau would receive this information, probably by telephone. When SPRINT is in operation, on-line input from the various municipal hospitals to the SPRINT computer can be considered. Extension of such an inventory system, where it does not yet exist, to nonmunicipal hospitals which provide emergency service would be encouraged.

INCREASED AVAILABILITY OF AMBULANCES

The simulation study showed that the combination of adding ambulances and shifting ambulances closer to the point of demand in a district produces improved service. The discussion here centers on low-cost means for increasing the effective use of available ambulances. The alternative of simply buying more ambulances is an obvious one that will be excluded from the discussion.

Improve Screening of Calls: About 15 percent of all calls turn out to be unnecessary, according to a recent statistical study of New York's emergency ambulance service.[3] More diligent efforts by personnel at the Communications Bureau to question the caller before deciding to dispatch an ambulance would reduce substantially the number of times that ambulances are sent out on unnecessary calls. (This is the procedure followed in Baltimore, Maryland, where only 8 percent of the calls turn out to be unnecessary.) By

[3] Dimendberg, D.C. "An Analysis of the Ambulance Service." New York, Department of Hospitals, 1967.

decreasing unnecessary ambulance utilization, service on true emergency calls will be improved.

Overtime Pay: Because drivers and attendants are not paid overtime rates, crews reportedly are reluctant to accept assignments a few minutes before their normal quitting time. If this is true, it would seem that the marginal cost of overtime labor might be an inexpensive way to buy more ambulances. In addition, by being able to offer overtime pay, an employee finishing one shift can be induced to work a second shift if his relief man fails to report to work; such absenteeism results in out-of-service ambulances.

Interchange of Crew Members: At present, ambulance attendants report to the nursing service in hospitals, while drivers are responsible to a garage foreman. This divided allegiance results in inflexible scheduling; for example, it is not possible to shift crews from one garage to another when there is a local shortage. Furthermore, if only a driver reports to work at one hospital, and only an attendant at another, pairing the two to provide one ambulance—instead of keeping two ambulances idle—is administratively awkward. By divorcing the ambulance service from the hospital itself, the resulting centralized authority over crew members should simplify the handling of such problems.

The suggestion also has been made that the same kind of training should be provided for both driver and attendant. This would permit complete interchangeability and, together with the change in policy on overtime pay, would result in fewer ambulances standing idle due to personnel absences.

Patient Acceptance Procedures: On certain classes of calls (for example, psychiatric cases), after delivering the patient, the ambulance crew must wait at the hospital for an inordinately long time before the ambulance is released and becomes available for reassignment. A change in the admission/acceptance procedure in such cases would increase the effective availability of ambulances.

Cost-Effectiveness Evaluation

EFFECTIVENESS

Average Response Time: Several simulation runs were conducted with ambulances stationed at various points in the district, for the purpose of comparing the proposed system of dispersed ambulances with the other

Table 19.

Average Response Time

	Number of Ambulances			
	7		*10*	
Alternatives	*Average Response Time*	*% Improve-ment*	*Average Response Time*	*% Improve-ment*
a. All Ambulances at Hospital	11.9'	0		
b. Optimal Allocation of Ambulances between Hospital and One Satellite	10.2'	14%	9.3'	22%
c. Totally Dispersed Ambulances	9.7'	18%	8.4'	30%

alternatives. The results are summarized in Table 19. It is clear that the dispersed system is superior to the other alternatives in terms of the improvement attainable; for example, 10 dispersed ambulances will reduce the response time by 30 percent (from the base case), whereas the same 10 ambulances distributed in optimal fashion (4/6) between hospital and satellite will produce only a 22-percent improvement. (Due to an adjustment in the mathematical model, the absolute values of the response times are not identical to the values shown on the figures and discussed earlier for identical ambulance configurations. This improvement does not change the earlier conclusions, nor does it alter significantly the percentage improvements.)

Reduction of Long Delays: The average response time in itself is insufficient to portray the effect of the alternatives on reducing the frequency of those unfortunate occurrences where a patient waits for an excessively long time before an ambulance appears. Because of the great desirability to reduce the fraction of calls which are subject to long delays, the effect of the alternatives on this factor also was examined. The findings are summarized in Table 20. Again, the dispersed pattern of operation is best by far:

Table 20.

Fraction of Calls with Response Time Greater Than Twenty Minutes

	Number of Ambulances			
	7		10	
Alternatives	*Fraction*	*% Improve-ment*	*Fraction*	*% Improve-ment*
a. All Ambulances at Hospital	.099	0		
b. Optimal Allocation of Ambulances Between Hospital and One Satellite	.073	26%	.051	48%
c. Totally Dispersed Ambulances	.065	34%	.03	69%

10 dispersed ambulances can be expected to reduce this fraction by 69 percent, compared to a 48-percent reduction with a satellite station. Inasmuch as mathematical models never duplicate the real world exactly, and because of statistical uncertainties in the findings, it is felt that although the absolute fractions of delayed calls (shown in Table 20) are not necessarily accurate, the relative improvements shown for the alternatives are indeed meaningful.

COSTS

The simulation results presented in the preceding section were devoted exclusively to portraying the effectiveness of the various alternatives. Now the costs must be examined. Table 21 displays the capital and operating costs for the various resources required. Using Table 22, which indicates the staffing patterns, the costs shown in Table 21 can be combined to reflect the incremental costs involved in going from the present configuration to each of the three alternative configurations; these are shown in Table 23.

Table 21.

Estimated Costs

	Purchase Price	Annual Cost	Total Annual Cost[a]
I. Vehicle (ambulance)	$5,700	$ 950	$ 950
Ambulance (6 yr. life)	4,900		
Equipment (6 yr. life)	800		
II. Vehicle (supervisory)		3,040	3,040
Sedan (2 yr. life)	2,000	1,000	
Equipment (5 yr. life)	200	40	
Maintenance and Supplies		2,000	
III. Vehicle Maintenance and Supplies		1,958	1,958
Maintenance and Repair Supplies		657	
Mechanics' Labor		505	
Gasoline and Oil		296	
Oxygen and Medical Supplies		500	
IV. Ambulance Crew		14,505	72,525
Motor Vehicle Operator		8,175	
Salary		6,500	
Overhead (22%)		1,430	
Uniform (allowance)		65	
Food Allowance		180	
Attendant		6,330	
Salary		5,000	
Overhead (22%)		1,100	
Uniform (issued)		50	
Food Allowance		180	
V. Garage		13,600	13,600
Rent		12,000	
Heat		1,100	
Light		300	
Telephone		200	
VI. Garage Staffing		14,516	72,580
Foreman		9,395	
Salary and Overhead		9,150	
Uniform and Food Allowance		245	
Clerk		5,121	
Salary and overhead		4,941	
Food Allowance		180	
VII. Cruising Supervisor		9,395	46,975

[a] For three shifts per day, seven days per week. Allowing for vacations, illnesses, etc., five crews are required to staff three shifts per day, seven days per week.

Table 22.

Deployment of Ambulances

Alternative	Tour 1		Tour 2		Tour 3		Total Number Ambulances in System	Additional Ambulances	Total Tours[a]	Added Tours
	E	T	E	T	E	T				
Seven ambulances (original pattern)	6	0	7	2	7	0	9	—	20	—
Eight ambulances	6	0	7	2	8	0	9	0	21	1
Nine ambulances	6	0	7	2	9	0	9	0	22	2
Ten ambulances	6	0	7	2	10	0	10	1	23	3

E = Emergency service   T = Transfer service
[a] Does not include transfer service.
Note: A tour is defined here as an 8-hour work period for each of seven days.

Table 23.

Incremental Costs of Alternatives

Alternative	Annual Cost	Monthly Cost
(A) 7 ambulances with a satellite	$ 86,180	$ 7,182
Garage	13,600	
Garage staffing	72,580	
(B) 10 ambulances with a satellite	161,613	13,468
Garage and garage staffing	86,180	
Additional ambulance	950	
Maintenance and supplies	1,958	
Ambulance crews (5)	72,525	
(C) 7 ambulances dispersed	16,700	1,400
Cruising supervisor and vehicle	16,700[a]	
(D) 8 ambulances dispersed	40,800	3,400
Cruising supervisor and vehicle	16,700[a]	
Ambulance crews (1⅔)	24,100	
(to staff one seven-day tour)		
(E) 9 ambulances dispersed	64,900	5,408
Cruising supervisor and vehicle	16,700[a]	
Ambulance crews (3⅓)	48,200	
(to staff two seven-day tours)		
(F) 10 ambulances dispersed	92,133	7,700
Cruising supervisor and vehicle	16,700[a]	
Additional ambulance	950	
Maintenance and supplies	1,958	
Ambulance crews (5)	72,525	
(to staff three seven-day tours)		

[a] Because a supervisor can cover 20–30 ambulances, a district of 7–10 ambulances requires only one-third of his time; hence, only one-third of the cost is charged to this district.
Note: The cost of a dispersed system does not include credit for savings due to staff, space, and equipment reductions at the base garage.

It is assumed that: on-the-street stations, with zero cost, are used for the dispersed ambulance systems; equivalent levels of supervision are employed for all alternatives, thus permitting accurate and fair comparisons to be made; and shift-to-shift staffing patterns are the same for each alternative, as shown in Table 22.

COST-EFFECTIVENESS

The cost-effectiveness of alternative ways of reducing response time and of reducing excessive delays is shown in Tables 24 and 25. The dramatic superiority of the dispersed configurations is self-evident; 8 dispersed ambulances (alternative D) are as effective as 10 ambulances in a satellite system (alternative B) at about one-fourth the incremental cost per call. This is a significant conclusion and a compelling argument for a dispersed system. Furthermore, the relative ranking of the alternatives is clear and unambiguous, even though the actual dollar figures in the cost-effectiveness columns of the tables may not be accurate enough for budgetary or accounting purposes. These tables give the policy maker the opportunity to make an enlightened choice as to the degree of improvement he wishes to aim for and the most efficient (least expensive) way to achieve that objective.

Table 24.

Cost-Effectiveness of Alternative Ways to Reduce Response Time

Alternative	*Effective-ness: Minutes Saved*	*Cost: $/Month*	*Cost-Effective-ness: $ per Minute*	*Cost per Call*
(A) 7 Ambulances with a Satellite	1.7	$ 7,182	$1.16	$1.96
(B) 10 Ambulances with a Satellite	2.6	13,468	1.42	3.68
(C) 7 Ambulances Dispersed	2.2	$ 1,400	.17	.38
(D) 8 Ambulances Dispersed	(2.6)	3,400	.36	.93
(E) 9 Ambulances Dispersed	(3.0)	5,408	.49	1.48
(F) 10 Ambulances Dispersed	3.5	7,700	.60	2.10

Note: Figures in parentheses are obtained by interpolation.

Table 25.

Cost-Effectiveness of Alternative Ways to Reduce Excessive Delays

Alternative	Effectiveness: Percentage Points Reduced Below 20 Minutes	Number Calls per Month Reduced Below 20 Minutes	Cost: $/Month	Cost Effectiveness: $ per Call Reduced
(A) 7 Ambulances with a Satellite	2.6	95	$ 7,182	$75.50
(B) 10 Ambulances with a Satellite	4.8	176	13,468	76.50
(C) 7 Ambulances Dispersed	3.4	125	1,400	11.20
(D) 8 Ambulances Dispersed	(4.6)	168	3,400	20.20
(E) 9 Ambulances Dispersed	(5.8)	222	5,408	24.40
(F) 10 Ambulances Dispersed	6.9	252	7,700	30.60

Note: Figures in parentheses are obtained by interpolation.

6

EVALUATION OF A FAMILY PLANNING
PROGRAM FOR AMERICAN INDIANS[1]

Introduction

During the period 1964–1965, the Division of Indian Health of the U.S. Public Health Service, which was responsible for providing health care to U.S. Indians and to Alaska natives, embarked on a significant expansion of its family planning services. After several years of operation, it conducted an evaluation of its family planning program to determine how efficient and effective it was.

Scope of the Evaluation

Essentially, the evaluation attempted to mesh the interests of economists and health administrators. Economists look upon family planning as a means for curbing the population explosion, reducing poverty, and relieving pressure on the economic resources of the country or the family. There is substantial evidence to support the assumption that lowering the birth rate will further these objectives. Thus, economists may consider that lowering the birth rate is a sufficient objective in itself.[2]

A health administrator, although he would agree with these objectives, has further objectives. Reducing the number of births, or the spacing of pregnancies, is viewed as a means of improving the health of mothers; but this is only part of the evaluation. This evaluation, conducted by health administrators, began with the assumption that the reduction in births, or the spacing

---

[1] This information was obtained from: Erwin S. Rabeau and Angel Reaud. "Evaluation of PHS Program Providing Family Planning Services for American Indians." Mimeographed paper presented before the Health Officers Section of the American Public Health Association at the Ninety-Sixth Annual Meeting, Detroit, Michigan, November 13, 1968.

[2] An economist also might be interested in the extent to which this lowered birth rate actually reduced poverty.

of pregnancies, would improve the health of the individual and of the community, although it was recognized that this assumption needed to be validated in the evaluation.

Objectives and Evaluation Criteria

In this evaluation, economists and medical administrators agreed that the principal objective of the family planning program was to cause the birth rate to decline, but medical administrators conducting the evaluation added further health status and health care objectives. They, therefore, set out to evaluate the following:

1. The extent to which the number of births and birth rates were reduced.
2. The extent to which health status and health care were improved.

They also sought to determine the costs of the programs.

Objective 1: Reduce the number of births and birth rates.
Evaluation Criteria: change in number of births, and change in birth rates.
This objective is attained primarily through contraception: by increasing the acceptance of contraception and the continuation of use upon acceptance. Thus, further clinical evaluation criteria are: extent of acceptance of contraception, and extent of continuation of contraceptive use. The evaluation, therefore, first addresses the extent of acceptance and the extent of continuation of contraceptive use and, finally, the specific reduction in births and birth rates.

Objective 2: Improved health care and health status.
In addition to reduction in births, an important objective for family planning programs is the improvement of health status and health care. This reflects certain assumptions made in the family planning process which are subject to validation through the evaluation process. In relation to the mother, the following is assumed:

1. The number of postpartum visits will increase, providing a better opportunity for the health supervision of the mother.

2. The spacing of pregnancies will provide more time for recovery after pregnancy and delivery, resulting in healthier mothers who will be less prone to pathologic (that is, difficult) pregnancies. This, in turn, will be reflected in decreased abortions, prematurity, and complications during pregnancy.

A basic tenet of family planning is that fewer children means healthier children. Thus, it is assumed that, in the long run, the family planning program will result in decreased infant morbidity and mortality. After several years of successful operation, benefits should be apparent in the older age groups (ages 1 to 4 and 5 to 14), because these older children, not being in competition with the newborn sibling, would receive more maternal care, would have better nutrition, and, as a consequence, would be in better health.

Validation of the above assumptions is not an easy task. Family planning programs, such as those operated by the Indian Health Service, tend to be a part of more comprehensive programs having a large number of activities affecting mothers and children. Isolation of these many variables, including family planning activities and determining their objective relationship to the changes in health status, requires a sophisticated use of analysis and of control groups. Such analysis has not been generally successful to date. In the absence of such sophistication, the following evaluation criteria are used:

1. Number of postpartum visits.
2. Number of abortions.
3. Percentage of premature births.
4. Pediatric[3] morbidity (as indicated by total days of pediatric hospitalization).
5. Infant mortality rate.

During the years analyzed (1960 to 1968), family planning was the only new program put in operation that was capable of affecting the trends in these indicators.

---

[3] Pediatric means children under 15 years of age.

Performance and Effectiveness

ACCEPTANCE

Acceptance refers to the proportion of women who could become pregnant (that is, proportion at risk) that begin contraception. Specifically, the population at risk of becoming pregnant is limited to fertile women that practice sexual relations; but, from a practical point of view, the target population or potential user group is the one of interest to the decision maker. Several groups may be defined.

1. The first, and largest, is the number of women of reproductive age (15 to 44 years) eligible for care.
2. The second, and smaller, group is the number of potential contraceptive users. This group can be determined by using the Polger Formula:[4] 17.8 percent of the population are women 18 to 44 years of age; of this number, 10 percent are nonfertile, therefore do not require birth control services. Of the fertile group eligible for care, 20 percent want to have children, leaving a balance of 80 percent as potential contraceptive users.
3. The third, and smallest, type of target population is the number of women hospitalized for delivery or abortion care during the period of the program.

The extent to which the program is accepted by these groups measures its selling characteristics, or the success of its efforts to interest couples to begin contraception. Following are the numbers of women in each group during fiscal year 1968:

1. Number of women of reproductive age—75,450.
2. Number of potential users of contraceptives—51,700.
3. Number of women hospitalized for delivery or abortion care—12,024 (11,176 cases of obstetrical delivery and 848 cases of abortion).

---

4 Jaffa, F. S. "Financing Family Planning Services." *American Journal of Public Health,* 56:912–917, June 1966.

ACCEPTANCE BY WOMEN OF REPRODUCTIVE AGE

During fiscal years 1962 and 1963, birth control services were limited, and detailed records were not kept. During fiscal year 1964, services were increased and programs were actively promoted, but accurate or comprehensive data are not available; specific reporting started in 1965.

Rather than attempting to reach all of the women of reproductive age, an immediate objective was set to reach 18,000 women, representing approximately 24 percent of the total. This figure was equivalent to the number of births expected at the prevailing birth rates for Indians and Alaska natives.

ACCEPTANCE BY POTENTIAL USERS

Table 26 shows the number of acceptors that started birth control and the cumulative number of acceptors, irrespective of duration of contraceptive use. Table 27 shows additional information of clinical interest: number of acceptors by method of contraception.

Table 26.

Family Planning Services Acceptance of the Program

Fiscal Year	New Acceptors	Cumulative Number of Acceptors[a]	Cumulative Number of Acceptors —Percent of Women 15 to 44 Years of Age
1968	6,610	21,477	28.5
1967	8,227	14,867	20.4
1966	2,779	6,640	9.2
1965	3,861	3,861	5.4

[a] Since inception of the program in fiscal year 1965.

Table 27.

Cumulative Number of Acceptors by Method of Contraception

Fiscal Year	Total Cumula- tive	Oral Contra- ceptives	Per- cent of Total	IUD's	Per- cent of Total	Other[a]	Per- cent of Total
1968	21,477	14,148	66.0	6,460	30.0	869	4.0
1967	14,867	9,423	63.4	4,734	31.8	710[b]	4.8
1966	6,640	4,641	69.9	1,999	30.1	NA	
1965	3,861	2,637	68.3	1,224	31.7	NA	

[a] Includes rhythm method, diaphragm, foam.
[b] Represents some carry-over from previous two years.

The cumulative number of new acceptors of reproductive age since July 1964 (fiscal year 1965) was 21,477 (28.5 percent). This was regarded as more than 100 percent of the immediate objective (18,000) to be reached.[5] Further information of operational interest is the number of women to whom contraceptive services were provided and the number of visits to physicians: 11,236 and 23,883 respectively in fiscal years 1967 and 1968.[6] Rather than helping to evaluate program effectiveness, however, such data are most useful in determining workloads for use in operational planning.

ACCEPTANCE BY WOMEN HOSPITALIZED FOR PREGNANCY OR ABORTION CARE
A review of patient records (those discharged after delivery or abortion) was conducted for the six-months period July 1 to December 31, 1967, in 25 Division of Indian Health Hospitals with more than 100 deliveries per year (a sample of 29 such hospitals). Instructions and services in family planning were offered to all of the aforementioned patients. Of the 3,696

[5] The evaluation did not consider reducing the cumulative number of acceptors by the number who discontinued use. Thus the figure does not represent a current count of women of reproductive age actually using contraceptive devices.
[6] There is undoubtedly some underreporting, because family planning is offered as part of a comprehensive health care program rather than in special family planning clinics. Data collection therefore is difficult. In addition, some such services are provided in family planning clinics operated by state and local authorities and are not included.

discharges, 1,448 women—representing 39 percent of the specific target population—accepted birth control services while in the hospital or within two months after discharge.[7]

A sample of 433 of the 572 women discharged from the same 25 hospitals during the month of December 1967 were interviewed in July 1968. The survey showed that 200 of the 433 women initiated contraception while in the hospital or within two months after discharge; 25 accepted contraceptive services two to six months after discharge. This shows an acceptance of 46 percent in the two months postpartum or postabortion period and an additional 6 percent two to six months after discharge.[8] Table 28 shows further data of clinical interest regarding the population served—age, marital status, and parity of the 9,552 women admitted to birth control service between February 1967 and July 1968.

CONTINUATION OF USE

The percentage of women that continued using the two major contraceptive methods was estimated. Because no specific study had been done on these patients, clinical impressions were used and compared to two known studies. It was estimated (Table 29) that the cumulative rates of expulsions, removals, and pregnancies for women using intrauterine devices (IUD's) were *approximately* those found in one analysis and *definitely lower* than those found in another.

With respect to oral contraceptives (pills), a study was conducted in the Public Health Service hospital in Tuba City, Arizona. Four hundred fifty-nine patients were started on oral contraceptives and followed up for 20 months. One hundred ninety women (42.5 percent) discontinued treatment after 1 to 13 months of contraception.[9] This compared to a drop-out rate of 10 percent for all races in the United States.

---

[7] These results were compared to those of the international postpartum family planning program, organized by the Population Council in 14 countries, which showed: U.S. hospitals, 45 percent; hospitals in other countries, 18 percent.

[8] Clinicians are interested in the fact that the method of contraception chosen by the 200 acceptors was: pills, 65 percent; IUD's, 31 percent; rhythm method, 2 percent; other methods, 2 percent. The method chosen by the acceptors of the two-to-six-months-after-discharge group was: pills, 64 percent; IUD's, 36 percent.

[9] Included in the 190 women were 5 who underwent sterilization operative procedures and 12 who changed to different methods of contraception. Of the remaining 173 (37.8 percent), 131 were lost to the program (presumably not heard from) and 42 discontinued contraception for medical or personal reasons.

Table 28.
Birth Control Services Provided to 9,552 Women Beneficiaries by Age, Marital Status, and Previous Number of Children Delivered

Age Group	Number of Women (new cases)	Married	Nonmarried	Unspecified	Number of New Cases in the Age Group According to the Previous Number of Children Delivered — Children Delivered Before Starting Birth Control														
					0	1	2	3	4	5	6	7	8	9	10	11	12	More Than 12	Unspecified
15–19	1,127	804	298	25	230	619	218	48	10	4									
20–24	2,922	2,359	376	187	160	800	856	600	329	121	29	17	3	5					6
25–29	2,477	2,042	232	203	99	234	405	549	510	324	218	118	53	22	6	2	1		4
30–34	1,532	1,310	103	119	18	32	114	161	245	265	206	186	131	93	41	21	10	9	1
35–39	885	763	59	63	4	14	34	45	68	84	103	107	106	92	77	63	32	47	
40–44	463	416	25	22	5	9	14	25	41	51	51	40	38	38	39	30	31	47	2
45 and over	126	121	5		2	3	7	8	10	12	11	13	8	8	12	6	7	16	
Unspecified	20	2		18								1							19
All Ages	9,552	7,817	1,098	637	518	1,711	1,648	1,436	1,213	861	618	482	311	258	175	122	81	119	32

Table 29.

Cumulative Rates of Events During First Year of
Intrauterine Loop Device—Three Studies

Event	*(1)* %	*(2)* %	*(3)* %
Expulsion	9.3	5–10	15.1
Removals	15.6	10–20	23.3
Pregnancies	2.4	2–3	3.2

(1) Data on 11,222 first insertions analyzed by the National Committee on Maternal Health.
(2) Division of Indian Health. Clinical impression.
(3) Emory University Family Planning Program. Grady Memorial Hospital. Study of 721 women.

The previously mentioned study of patients discharged during December 1968 showed that, six months after discharge, 151 of 200 (76 percent) women interviewed who accepted birth control during the two months postpartum or postabortion period were practicing contraception.[10]

NUMBER OF BIRTHS AVERTED AND QUANTITATIVE REDUCTION OF BIRTHS
AND BIRTH RATES

Although nearly everyone agrees that it is reasonable to expect that a family planning program should result in lowered birth rates, no one knows precisely (or even approximately) what the quantity of the relationship should be. Table 30 shows the trend in birth rates for Indians and Alaska

Table 30.

Live Births: Division of Indian Health Hospitals

Fiscal Year	Indians	Alaska Natives	Total	Percent of Change
1967	7,424	1,121	8,545	−7.6
1966	8,046	1,197	9,243	−4.9
1965	8,643	1,076	9,719	+0.3
1964	8,612	1,075	9,687	+3.5
1963	8,334	1,026	9,360	+2.9
1962	8,205	889	9,094	+5.3
1961	7,811	824	8,635	+1.3
1960	7,693	826	8,519	—

[10] This includes all methods, and the data are not broken out by type of contraception.

natives for fiscal years 1960 to 1967. The number of births increased steadily until 1965, when there was a leveling off. In fiscal years 1966 and 1967, there were reductions of 4.9 and 7.6 percent respectively. Such data are least subject to distortion by fluctuations in population when expressed in terms of birth rates[11] and fertility rates.[12] Table 31 shows these birth and fertility rates from 1960 to 1966 (the last year for which data were available) for Indians, Alaska natives, and United States—all races.

Clearly, the birth rates for Indians and Alaska natives were increasing until 1964 and then began to decline dramatically. Although it cannot be proven that the family planning program was directly responsible for this reduction, it has been scientifically proven that contraception can be effective in lowering the birth rates.[13]

Other Health Care and Health Status Measures

POSTPARTUM VISITS

The usual experience elsewhere has been that the inception of a family planning program for obstetrical patients immediately produces an increase in the number of six-week, postpartum visits. In the Indian Health Programs, the average number of postpartum visits per year for 1961 to 1963 was 3,236; the average for 1965 to 1967 increased by 64 percent to 5,315 visits per year.

ABORTIONS

If the family planning program is effective, the number of abortions must decrease. The number of abortion patients admitted to hospitals decreased by 20 percent from 1965 to 1967 (1,071 patients were admitted in 1965 versus 848 in 1967).

---

[11] The number of live births per 1,000 population.

[12] The number of live births per 1,000 women age 15 to 44.

[13] It seems reasonable to attribute at least a large portion of the reduction to the program. Referring again to the survey of 433 women interviewed in July 1968 who were discharged due to delivery or abortion in December 1967, there were 225 who accepted birth control services within six months of discharge and 208 who did not. By this time (six months after discharge), 3.5 percent of the first group were pregnant versus 10.5 percent of the second group.

Table 31.

Birth Rate and Fertility Rate: Indians, Alaska Natives, and United States—all Races

Calendar Year	Birth Rate[a]				Fertiliy Rate[b]			
	Indians	Alaska Natives	Indians and Alaska Natives	U.S.—All Races	Indians	Alaska Natives	Indians and Alaska Natives	U.S.—All Races
1966	38.5	41.1	38.7	18.4	204.9	218.4	206.0	91.3
1965	41.5	43.4	41.7	19.4	220.9	230.8	221.8	96.6
1964	43.1	45.7	43.3	21.0	229.0	243.1	230.2	105.0
1963	42.4	49.5	43.0	21.7	225.4	263.1	228.6	108.5
1962	42.1	48.6	42.7	22.4	224.0	258.7	226.9	112.2
1961	42.3	48.6	42.8	23.3	225.1	258.4	227.9	117.2
1960	42.2	45.6	42.5	23.7	224.3	242.6	225.9	118.0

[a] Number of live births per 1000 population.
[b] Number of live births per 1000 women 15 to 44 years of age.

PREMATURITY (BIRTH WEIGHT 2,500 GRAMS OR LESS)

The percentage of premature births increased slightly every year from 1962 to 1964 (6.0, 7.1, and 7.4 percent respectively). From 1965 to 1967, it declined 6.8, 6.7, and 6.2 percent respectively.

PEDIATRIC MORBIDITY

Table 32 shows the number of days of hospitalization of children under 15 years of age from 1960 to 1967, as indicated in the evaluation. A definite increasing trend was shown to 1964, when it began to decline. A better presentation would have been the rate of hospitalization per 1,000 children under 15 years of age. We cannot tell from these data what the change in population base might have been.

Table 32.

Total Days of Hospitalization, Children under 15 Years of Age:
Division of Indian Health Hospital

Fiscal Year	*Days of Hospitalization*
1967	228,077
1966	243,797
1965	242,996
1964	271,766
1963	261,521
1962	249,172
1961	221,159
1960	211,273

INFANT MORTALITY

It is particularly difficult to interpret the change in the infant mortality rate, which had been declining prior to the initiation of the family planning program. Based on the data in Table 33, it is difficult to establish a correlation between birth control and decrease in infant mortality. The infant mortality rate throughout the country, as well as for Indians and Alaska natives, had been declining steadily for several years. The lowest rate for Indians and Alaska natives was in 1964, with the rate increasing somewhat thereafter.

Table 33.

Infant Mortality Rate (Per 1,000 Live Births):
Indians, Alaska Natives, and U.S.—All Races

Fiscal Year	Indians	Alaska Natives	Indians and Alaska Natives	U.S.— All Races
1966	37.7	51.4	39.0	23.7
1965	36.4	65.4	39.0	24.7
1964	35.9	54.8	37.6	24.8
1963	42.9	50.7	43.6	25.2
1962	41.8	66.8	44.2	25.3
1961	42.3	64.0	44.4	25.3
1960	47.6	76.3	50.3	26.0

Cost Analysis

The cost of a family planning program, when it is part of a more comprehensive health program such as that provided by the Division of Indian Health, is difficult to estimate with precision. Family planning activities in such settings are only one element of the total comprehensive health program, and, often, budget-line items for such services are not maintained. Such services are commonly provided through general medical and surgical clinics, gynecology and obstetrics clinics, or postpartum clinics. Accordingly, cost figures used in this evaluation are only rough estimates. The Division did, however, keep estimates (on a monthly basis) of expenditures for the following: oral contraceptives; intrauterine devices; contract physicians' fees; contraceptive drugs prescribed by contract physicians; and pamphlets, films, posters, etc.

It was therefore known that oral contraceptives at government prices had an average cost of about $0.60 for one month's supply and, when prescribed by contract physicians and purchased at a retail drug store, that the average cost for one month's supply was about $2.25. Intrauterine devices had an average cost of about $1.00 per device at government prices.

The above cost elements are relatively straightforward, and it was possible to estimate costs directly from the program's records. An important element of cost, however, includes the time devoted to family planning services by the Division staff—physicians, pharmacists, nurses, social workers, health educators, and administrative and clerical help. Rather than attempt to determine the true incremental costs of this particular program, which was thought to be impossible to separate from other functions, it was decided to determine a fully allocated cost that would be roughly equivalent to a price charged for the service. These expenditures were estimated to be $3.89 (1967) and $3.36 (1968) for each outpatient visit, exclusive of drugs and devices. These expenditures include costs for a physician, clinic nurse, pharmacist, administrative and clerical help, and housekeeping, but exclude amortization and depreciation of facilities and equipment. The costs of other personnel services were determined by estimating the percentage of total time devoted to family planning activities by nurses, social workers, and health educators, plus an allowance for administrative and clerical support. It was estimated that each spent about 2.5 percent of his total time in family planning activities. Recognizing the shortcomings of this approach and the fact that it does not truly represent an incremental cost, nevertheless, Table 34 depicts the family planning program costs as determined in the evaluation.

In 1967, 12,506 women (including both new and previous acceptors) received birth control services, at a total cost of $268,000. This represents a cost of about $21 per woman. In 1968, 11,236 women were provided services, at a total cost of $275,000 or about $24 per woman. If the estimated

Table 34.

Family Planning Program Costs—Fiscal Years 1967 and 1968
(In Thousands of Dollars)

Cost Category	Fiscal Year	
	1967	*1968*
Drugs and Intrauterine Devices	43.9	55.1
Visits to Indian Health Division Physicians	117.4	95.0
Contract Physicians' Fees	1.9	5.0
Public Health Nurses, Social Workers, and Health Educators	97.0	108.0
Films, Pamphlets, Posters	7.8	11.9
TOTAL	*268.0*	*275.0*

expenditures for Public Health nurses, health educators, and social workers were excluded from the total figures to permit comparisons with other programs, the cost per woman provided services in 1967 and 1968 was $14 and $15 respectively. This figure compares favorably with the estimated total annual cost of $26 (including direct and definable indirect costs) per acceptor in U. S. hospitals in 1967.[14]

Implications and Conclusions

The evaluation indicates some substantial benefits of the family planning programs being evaluated. It should be persuasive to physicians because of its clinical criteria, as well as to other types of evaluators and decision makers because of its quantitative evaluation criteria.

In terms of the criterion of acceptance, the statistics are most impressive. Nearly 29 percent of the women of reproductive age started birth control measures. Similarly, nearly one-half ‘of the women discharged from hospitals due to pregnancy or abortion care accepted birth control services. Clearly, a significant reduction in births and birth rates was achieved beginning with the inception of the program. A large portion of the reduction can be attributed to the family planning program. Significant improvements also were made in other health care and health status measures, including postpartum visits, abortions, prematurity, and infant mortality. The costs of the program compare quite favorably with the costs of other family planning programs.

This study presents the decision maker with a clear, overwhelming mass of evidence which shows that the program apparently is achieving its objectives in a cost-effective manner. The program has been continued and expanded since the evaluation was conducted.

[14] This estimate was made by the Population Council, International Family Planning Program. Ideally, the costs should be adjusted to reflect inflation from 1967 to 1968.

APPENDIX

Comprehensive Health Center Structure

		Investment $	Time in Operation	Operating $ 1st Year	$/Month	Annual Operating Cost
11.	ADMINISTRA-TIVE					
.1	Personnel					
.11	Professional					
.12	Technical					
.13	Support					
.14	Adm. Contract					
.2	Fringe Benefits					
.5	Equipment					
.51	Permanent					
.511	Facility					
.52	Consumable					
.6	Travel					
.7	Maintenance					
.9	Miscellaneous					
12.	MEDICAL SERVICES					
.1	Personnel					
.11	Professional					
.12	Technical					
.13	Support					
.5	Equipment					
.51	Permanent					
.52	Consumable					
.6	Travel					
.7	Referral					
.8	Hospitalization					
.9	Miscellaneous					

	Investment $	Time in Operation	Operating $ 1st Year	$/Month	Annual Operating Cost
13. **CONSUL-TANTS & CONTRACTS**					
.1 Personnel					
.11 Professional					
.12 Technical					
.13 Support					
.5 Equipment					
.51 Permanent					
.52 Consumable					
.6 Travel					
.8 Hospitalization					
.9 Miscellaneous					
14. **OB/GYN**					
.1 Personnel					
.11 Professional					
.12 Technical					
.13 Support					
.5 Equipment					
.51 Permanent					
.52 Consumable					
.6 Travel					
.8 Hospitalization					
.9 Miscellaneous					
15. **PEDIATRICS**					
.1 Personnel					
.11 Professional					
.12 Technical					
.13 Support					
.5 Equipment					
.51 Permanent					
.52 Consumable					
.6 Transportation					
.8 Hospitalization					
.9 Miscellaneous					
16. **INTERNAL MEDICINE**					
.1 Personnel					
.11 Professional					
.12 Technical					
.13 Support					

	Investment $	Time in Operation	Operating $ 1st Year	$/Month	Annual Operating Cost
.5 Equipment					
.51 Permanent					
.52 Consumable					
.6 Transportation					
.8 Hospitalization					
.9 Miscellaneous					
17. GENERAL PRACTICE					
.1 Personnel					
.11 Professional					
.12 Technical					
.13 Support					
.5 Equipment					
.51 Permanent					
.52 Consumable					
.6 Travel					
.8 Hospitalization					
.9 Miscellaneous					
18. MENTAL HEALTH					
.1 Personnel					
.11 Professional					
.12 Technical					
.13 Support					
.5 Equipment					
.51 Permanent					
.52 Consumable					
.6 Travel					
.8 Hospitalization					
.9 Miscellaneous					
19. RADIOLOGY					
.1 Personnel					
.11 Professional					
.12 Technical					
.13 Support					
.5 Equipment					
.51 Permanent					
.52 Consumable					
.6 Travel					
.8 Hospitalization					
.9 Miscellaneous					

	Investment $	Time in Operation	Operating $ 1st Year	$/Month	Annual Operating Cost
20. **PHARMACY**					
.1 Personnel					
.11 Professional					
.12 Technical					
.13 Support					
.5 Equipment					
.51 Permanent					
.52 Consumable					
.6 Travel					
.9 Miscellaneous					
21. **LABORATORY**					
.1 Personnel					
.11 Professional					
.12 Technical					
.13 Support					
.5 Equipment					
.51 Permanent					
.52 Consumable					
.6 Travel					
.7 Special Tests					
.8 Sterilization					
.9 Miscellaneous					
22. **DENTAL**					
.1 Personnel					
.11 Professional					
.12 Technical					
.13 Support					
.5 Equipment					
.51 Permanent					
.52 Consumable					
.9 Miscellaneous					
23. **COMMUNITY ACTION**					
.1 Personnel					
.11 Professional					
.12 Technical					
.13 Support					
.2 Rehabilitation					
.21 Personnel					
.22 Equipment					
.5 Equipment					

		Investment $	Time in Operation	Operating $ 1st Year	$/Month	Annual Operating Cost
.51	Permanent					
.52	Consumable					
.6	Travel					
.9	Miscellaneous					
24.	MANPOWER					
.1	Personnel					
.11	Professional					
.12	Technical					
.13	Support					
.14	Trainees					
.5	Equipment					
.51	Permanent					
.52	Consumable					
.6	Travel					
.9	Miscellaneous					
25.	SATELLITE UNIT					
.1	Personnel					
.11	Professional					
.12	Technical					
.13	Support					
.5	Equipment					
.51	Permanent					
.52	Consumable					
.6	Travel					
.8	Referral					
.9	Miscellaneous					
26.	PROGRAM EVALUATION					
.1	Personnel					
.11	Professional					
.12	Technical					
.13	Support					
.5	Equipment					
.51	Permanent					
.52	Consumable					
.6	Travel					
.7	Computer Time					
.9	Miscellaneous					

BIBLIOGRAPHY

BOOKS AND MONOGRAPHS

Arrow, K. J. *Social Choice and Individual Value.* Cowles Commission Monograph No. 12. New York, Wiley, 1951.

Bauer, Raymond, ed. *Social Indicators.* Cambridge, Mass., M.I.T. Press, 1966.

Bauer, Raymond and Gergen, Kenneth J. *The Study of Policy Formulation.* New York, Free Press, 1968.

Black, Guy. *The Application of Systems Analysis to Government Operations.* New York, Praeger, 1968.

Buchanan, James M. *Public Finance in Democratic Process.* Chapel Hill, University of North Carolina Press, 1967.

Buchanan, James and Tullock, Gordon. *The Calculus of Consent: Logical Foundations of Constitutional Democracy.* Ann Arbor, University of Michigan Press, 1962.

Burkhead, Jesse. *Government Budgeting.* New York, Wiley, 1956.

Burt, Marvin R. et al. *Delivery and Financing of Health Services to the Poor: A Cost-Effectiveness Analysis.* Bethesda, Md., Resource Management Corp., 1967.

Chase, Samuel B., ed. *Problems in Public Expenditure Analysis.* Washington, D.C., The Brookings Institution, 1968.

Dahl, Robert. *A Preface to Democratic Theory.* Chicago, University of Chicago Press, 1956.

DonVito, P. A. *Annotated Bibliography in Systems Cost Analysis.* Santa Monica, Calif., The RAND Corporation, 1968. RM 4848-PR.

Dorfman, Robert, ed. *Measuring Benefits of Government Investments.* Washington, D.C., The Brookings Institution, 1965.

Downs, Anthony. *An Economic Theory of Democracy.* New York, Harper, 1957.

Dror, Yehezkel. *Public Policymaking Re-examined.* San Francisco, Chandler, 1968.

Fein, Rashi. *The Doctor Shortage.* Washington, D.C., The Brookings Institution, 1967.

Feldstein, Paul J. *An Empirical Investigation of the Marginal Cost of Hospital Services.* Chicago, Graduate Program in Hospital Administration, University of Chicago, 1961.

127

Fishburn, Peter C. *Decision and Value Theory.* New York, Wiley, 1964.

Frankel, Charles. *The Case for Modern Man.* New York, Harper, 1956.

Gass, Saul I. *Linear Programming.* New York, McGraw-Hill, 1964.

Hatry, H. P. *The Use of Cost Estimates in Cost-Effectiveness Analysis.* Washington, D.C., Office of Assistant Secretary of Defense (Comptroller) Programming Office, 1965.

Hatry, Harry P. and Cotton, John F. *Program Planning for State-County-City.* Washington, D. C., The George Washington University, 1967.

Helmer, Olaf. *Social Technology.* New York, Basic Books, 1966.

Hitch, Charles and McKean, Roland. *The Economics of Defense in the Nuclear Age.* Cambridge, Mass., Harvard University Press, 1960.

Jones, M. V. *System Cost Analysis: A Management Tool for Decision Making.* Bedford, Mass., The MITRE Corporation, 1964. TM-4063.

Klarman, Herbert E. *The Economics of Health.* New York, Columbia University Press, 1965.

Large, J. P., ed. *Concepts and Procedures of Cost Analysis.* Santa Monica, Calif., The RAND Corporation, 1963.

Lindblom, C. E. *The Intelligence of Democracy.* New York, Free Press, 1965.

March, James G. and Simon, Herbert A. *Organizations.* New York, Wiley, 1958.

McKean, R. N. *Efficiency in Government Through Systems Analysis.* New York, Wiley, 1958.

Mishan, E. J. *Welfare Economics.* New York, Random House, 1964.

Musgrove, Richard A., ed. *Essays in Fiscal Federalism.* Washington, D.C., The Brookings Institution, 1965.

Novick, David, ed. *Program Budgeting: Program Analysis and the Federal Government.* Cambridge, Mass., Harvard University Press, 1965.

————. *System and Total Force Cost Analysis.* Santa Monica, Calif., The RAND Corporation, 1961. RM-2695.

Ott, David J. and Ott, Attiat F. *Federal Budget Policy.* Washington, D.C., The Brookings Institution, 1965.

Quade, E. S., ed. *Analysis for Military Decisions.* Santa Monica, Calif., The RAND Corporation, 1964.

Smithies, Arthur. *Government Decision-Making and the Theory of Choice.* Santa Monica, Calif., The RAND Corporation, 1964.

————. *The Budgetary Process in the United States.* New York, McGraw-Hill, 1955.

Simon, Herbert. *Administrative Behavior.* 2nd Ed. New York, Macmillan, 1957.

————. *Models of Man.* New York, Wiley, 1957.

Weidenbaum, Murray L. *Federal Budgeting: The Choice of Government Programs.* Washington, D.C., American Enterprise Institute, 1964.

Weisbrod, Burton A. *Economics of Public Health.* Philadelphia, University of Pennsylvania Press, 1961.

Wildavsky, Aaron. *The Politics of the Budgetary Process.* Boston, Little, Brown, 1964.

ARTICLES

Abert, James G. "Structuring Cost-Effectiveness Analysis." *Logistics Review and Military Logistics Journal, 11*(7):19–34, 1966.

Banks, Robert L. and Kotz, Arnold. "The Program Budget and the Interest Rate for Public Investment." *Public Administration Review, 26*(4):283–292, December 1966.

Bateman, Worth. "Assessing Program Effectiveness." *Welfare in Review*, January–February 1968, pp. 1–10.

Dror, Yehezkel. "Policy Analysts: A New Professional Role in Government Service." *Public Administration Review, 27*(3):197–203, September 1967.

Enthoven, Alain C. "Decision Theory and Systems Analysis." *Armed Forces Comptroller, 9*(1):12–17, 38–39, 1964.

Flagle, Charles. "Operations Research in the Health Services." *Operations Research, 10*(4):591–603, 1962.

Gorham, William. "Sharpening the Knife that Cuts the Public Pie." *Public Administration Review, 28*(3):236–241, May/June 1968.

Hertz, David. "Risk Analysis in Capital Investment." *Harvard Business Review, 42*(1):95–106, January/February 1964.

Hitch, Charles. "Suboptimization in Operations Research Problems." *Journal of the Operations Research Society of America, 1*(3):79–87, May 1953.

Key, V. O., Jr. "The Lack of a Budgetary Theory." *The American Political Science Review, 34*(4):1137–1144, 1940.

Lewis, Verne B. "Toward a Theory of Budgeting." *Public Administration Review, 12*(1):42–54, Winter 1952.

Mosher, Frederick C. "PPBS: Two Questions." *Public Administration Review, 27*(1):67–71, March 1967.

Packer, A. H. "Applying Cost-Effectiveness Concepts to the Community Health System." *Operations Research, 16*(2):227–254, March–April 1968.

Schick, Allen. "The Road to PPB: The Stages of Budget Reform." *Public Administration Review, 26*(4):243–258, December 1966.

Wildavsky, Aaron. "The Political Economy of Efficiency: Cost-Benefit Analysis, Systems Analysis, and Program Budgeting." *Public Administration Review, 26*(4):292–310, December 1966.

GOVERNMENT DOCUMENTS

Rice, Dorothy D. *Estimating the Cost of Illness.* U.S. Department of Health, Education, and Welfare. Health Economic Series, No. 6. Washington, D.C., U.S. Government Printing Office, 1966.

U.S. Department of Health, Education, and Welfare (Public Health Service). *Comprehensive Health Planning: A Selected Annotated Bibliography.* Washington, D.C., 1967.

————. *Disease Control Program: Arthritis.* Washington, D.C., Office of the Assistant Secretary for Program Coordination, 1966.

————. *Disease Control Programs: Cancer.* Washington, D.C., Office of the Assistant Secretary for Program Coordination, 1966.

————. *Kidney Disease Program Analysis.* Washington, D.C., U.S. Public Health Service, 1967.

————. *Disease Control Programs: Motor Vehicle Injury Prevention Program.* Washington, D.C., Office of the Assistant Secretary for Program Coordination, 1966.

————. *Disease Control Programs: Selected Disease Control Programs.* Washington, D.C., Office of the Assistant Secretary for Program Coordination, 1966.

————. *Human Investment Programs: Delivery of Health Services for the Poor.* Washington, D.C., U.S. Government Printing Office, 1967.

————. *Maternal and Child Health Care Programs.* Washington, D.C., Office of the Assistant Secretary for Program Coordination, 1966.

————. *Proceedings: Conference-Workshop on Regional Medical Programs.* 2 Vols. January 1968.

U.S. Government (Bureau of the Budget). *The Budget of the United States, 1969.* Washington, D.C., U.S. Government Printing Office, 1968.

————. *Special Analyses, Budget of the United States, 1969.* Washington, D.C., U.S. Government Printing Office, 1968.

AUTHOR INDEX

SUBJECT INDEX

Abortion rate
  in American Indians and Alaska natives, 114
A fortiori analysis, 10
Alaska natives
  evaluation of family planning program for, 53, 54, 105–119
Alternative disease control programs
  cost analysis, 43–45
Alternative health services programs
  cost analysis, 45–48
Alternatives
  delivery of health care, 33–35, 43–48
  emergency ambulance service, New York, 75, 101–103
  health program analysis, 15, 25, 43, 44, 64–65
  maternal and child health care programs, 64–65, 66–72
  selection of, 25, 43, 45–48
Ambulance service, *see* Emergency ambulance service, New York
American Indians
  evaluation of family planning program for, 53, 54, 105–119
Analysis
  a fortiori, 10
  contingency, 10
  program, 9
  sensitivity, 10
  see also Cost analysis
  see also Health program analysis
  see also Policy analysis
Analysis for Military Decisions, 29
"An Analysis of the Ambulance Service," 95
Annotated Bibliography on Systems Cost Analysis, 29

"Applying Cost-Effectiveness Concepts to the Community Health System," 19, 27, 28, 39, 42, 44

Benefit-cost analysis, *see* Cost analysis
A Benefit-Cost Analysis of Maternal and Child Health Care Programs, 71
Birth rate
  of American Indians and Alaska natives, 106, 113–114, 115

Cardinal utility theory, 40, 42
Case-finding programs, 64–65
Child health needs, 57–59
Children's Bureau, 61
Chronic disease
  in children, 60, 61, 62, 68
Communication subsystem
  emergency medical care, 74, 92–93, 95–96
Comprehensive health care
  cost analysis, 38, 46–48
  estimated program effectiveness, 32
  maternal and child health care programs, 64, 66–72
  model of center structure, 121–125
  need for, 21, 23
Computer simulation
  emergency ambulance service, New York, 79–83
Concepts and Procedures of Cost Analysis, 29
Concepts and Techniques for Summarizing Defense System Costs, 29
Conceptual Problems in Developing an Index of Health, 19
Consumer Price Index (CPI), 30
Contingency analysis, 10